The Integral Being

J. A. Yaryura-Tobias, M.D.

The Integral Being

A NEW PATH TO PERSONAL GROWTH AND MEANINGFUL LIVING

Henry Holt and Company   *New York*

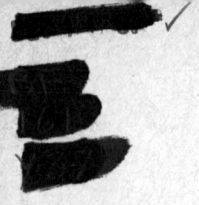

Copyright © 1987 by J. A. Yaryura-Tobias
All rights reserved, including the right to reproduce
this book or portions thereof in any form.
Published by Henry Holt and Company, Inc.,
521 Fifth Avenue, New York, New York 10175.
Published in Canada by Fitzhenry & Whiteside Limited,
195 Allstate Parkway, Markham, Ontario L3R 4T8.

Library of Congress Cataloging in Publication Data
Yaryura-Tobias, Jose A., 1934–
The integral being.
1. Mind and body. 2. Emotions. 3. Health.
4. Healing. I. Title.
BF161.Y37 1987   158   86-33563
ISBN 0-8050-0101-8

First Edition

Designer: Victoria Hartman
Printed in the United States of America
1 3 5 7 9 10 8 6 4 2

For those who believe in freedom and mutual respect

Contents

Acknowledgments ix
INTRODUCTION 1
1 · COSMIC INTEGRATION 11
2 · THE FAMILY 23
3 · SOCIETY 38
4 · GOVERNMENT 49
5 · THE SMALL TRIANGLE 64
6 · THE BODY 76
7 · THE PASSIONS 93
8 · THE INTELLECT 119
9 · ON DISEASE 135
10 · THE ART OF HEALING 146
11 · THE ART OF PREVENTION 159
12 · WE AND THE BEYOND 177
13 · THE ONGOING YOU 185
EPILOGUE 195

Acknowledgments

To my editors Richard Seaver and Channa Taub, I feel grateful for their having taught me how to distinguish between what I wrote and what I thought I wrote. Happily I was surrounded by enthusiastic friends who gave me support all along. Among them, Larry and Jean Fornasieri, and Beth Forhman. Special appreciation to my Renaissance friend Fred Penzel—busiest among the busiest—who set aside many hours of his time to help me out with the book. My gratitude goes also to my wife and children, who had the patience to listen to the readings of my chapters and to my dreams about the book. I know they stoically tolerated my isolation and frustration. They sensed and understood my feelings when things did not go as expected. My appreciation to my secretary Dolores Barry, who tirelessly retyped the manuscript. And special recognition to my daughter Ana Maria, who suggested the title *The Integral Being,* in lieu of "The Integral Man," as the best way to integrate men, women, and children from the start.

The Integral Being

INTRODUCTION

> The man who regards his own life and that of his fellow creatures as meaningless is not merely unhappy but hardly fit for life.
>
> Albert Einstein, "The Meaning of Life" (1934) from *Ideas and Opinions* (1954)

I have been told I was born on top of the desk in my uncle's medical office, in answer perhaps to my grandmother, who once said, "I had fifteen children born at home." Bringing me into the universe, in 1934, required the obstetrician to use forceps. Clear evidence, even then, of my perennial inability to accept orders I consider unjust—not having been consulted or informed, I was unwilling to be born. Later, when I was ten years old, my mother died. Again, I was not consulted. At ten I regarded her death as unfair, and, in my many years as a physician, I have not changed my views on death.

I have been a son, a brother, a husband, a father, a dreamer, a rebel, a poet, a writer, an internist, a psychiatrist, a scientist, a citizen, and an immigrant. Yet, who am I?

I am constantly amazed by life and nature. I have experienced success and failure, courage and fear. I have been betrayed, ignored, lied to, unwanted, scorned, supported, helped, understood, loved, and hated. I care for my fellow beings because I, too, need to be cared for. At times I feel discouraged at being alive, with suffering so long and happiness just a mere coffee break that most of us miss. Yet I never give up.

I was educated in Argentina under Perón's regime. I quickly became aware of social injustice, oppression, and the exploitation of man by man, not only in my own country but all over the world. No matter where we live, however, we are deprived of freedom. We admire the success of the corrupted, worship the power of the ruler, and envy the wealth of the exploiter. We are outraged if a dog is mistreated but are quiet about the existence of political torture. Violence is rampant and democracy, if it exists, is relative. Family is in question, food is artificial, water is contaminated, air lacks oxygen. We are no longer individuals but clusters of confused puppets grasping for courage.

We have enough technology to feed several planets, yet famine is commonplace. We can transplant organs to delay death, yet we have built enough bombs to displace the earth from its orbit. Time is running out for us. Therefore, it is imperative that we change.

We need not live in trepidation and uncertainty, haunted by fear of war or hunger, of getting old, or longing to be accepted and loved. We can live happily, in peace and in freedom.

Must we change to do this? Certainly not, if we feel content with our life-style, if we live in a social environment of justice and freedom. But if we are restless, under stress, drinking or using drugs to escape reality, if we find life worthless, if we have become spectators rather than participants in life, then we'd better do something about it.

We all have a world ready to be discovered, a world that

can be turned on to fill our needs, a world that will speak the language of our feelings, a world of understanding and acceptance of who we are, of what we do, a world that will accept us with our virtues and our defects.

After birth, we are constantly shattered from within and without. Our bodies, emotions, reasoning, families, the communities in which we live—nature in general—seem not to be part of the whole of the universe. Somewhere, sometime in the history of mankind, or perhaps even in our personal histories, we began a process of detachment from the universe. My experience as a man and as a psychiatrist has continuously exposed me to pain and despair, at times difficult to soothe. Because I have witnessed so many failures, my own and others, it has forced me to seek new explanations once the conventional resources were exhausted.

For instance, I could treat patients for depression, prescribe the right medication, help to change negative attitudes, and bring some humor into their lives; nonetheless, there was always something missing. I could meet a friend I hadn't seen for many years; everything was fine—family, work, success—yet I would sense an emptiness, a subtle aging in a man still young. So I began to search, started to read more, went back to history, to the saga of the creation of the modern world. Consequently, I came to the realization that to be *integral* was the solution to existence. This answer is not a new one; suggestions of it are evident in Eastern philosophies, in many religions, and in Mayan history.

The definition of *integral* is "lacking nothing that belongs to it." Therefore, becoming integral would improve our lives by filling in the empty spaces, that is, living in harmony with our internal and external environment. In this way, integral beings can maintain their health, defend their freedom, and preserve their individuality.

To become integral beings we have to follow an integral approach. This means learning more about the external systems we live in and their interplay with our internal systems. The human body is continuously bombarded by external stimuli of physical or psychosocial origin that reach the brain. Subsequently, the brain has to analyze and dispose of these messages in order to execute appropriate responses. From a biological viewpoint, all of this activity is geared to maintain our equilibrium with outside elements, for the ultimate purpose of survival. But having decided to become integral beings, our purpose goes beyond survival—we need to strive to live in peace and harmony.

We should become acquainted with history to understand how things evolved. History not only means knowledge about past societies and facts about our ancestors, but also whether we were breast- or bottle-fed. Without knowing the systems that formed us we cannot function.

Integral beings also must learn to be responsible for their thoughts and actions. This responsibility cannot be shared. Historically, mankind has had a propensity to attribute natural events to individuals or divine entities. Instead of entertaining the idea of a group brainstorming the whole process of the creation, most religions have chosen one divine being. Consequently, we have made gods responsible for the universe, as well as for our thoughts and actions. This assumption gives us the right to blame someone else for our wrongdoings. Although this may sound like an overture to rejecting the idea of God, it is actually an invitation to accept the idea of our own divinity.

Let us speculate that one day a snapshot of God can be taken. This event will dispute the theological invisibility of

God. As a consequence, the credibility of God may decline. But a new visibility, the materialization of God, will occur. At this point, the existing disparity between matter and spirit will be resolved, opening the gates to a new world of understanding and tolerance—the world of the integral being.

In the meantime, we should become integral beings to fulfill our aims, and progress within nature. Eventually we will begin to reap the benefits: tranquillity, acquisition, fulfillment of dreams. Hard work is, of course, not only required but expected. And we must tackle problems with reason and passion, wisdom and humility.

The integral being is one who is proud of existing on earth not to collect but to share, not to rule but to suggest, not to offend but to respect. These attitudes and behaviors are contagious for those whose spirits and minds are ready to unfold their hidden potentials, to reach a new and positive dimension, and to enhance the earth where we dwell.

Where do I come from?
What is the purpose of my life?
Who am I?

I think of myself as a cell orbiting outside the universe, floating alone in infinite darkness. Then one day I start my journey to Earth. Along the way I pick up more cells, colors, smells, emotions, intelligence, a face. I witness the stars and the planets, the traveling lights, the black holes. . . . I am drawn into dimensions I may never experience again. Finally, I arrive on Earth. I am a composite of fire, air, water, and soil. I will burn and blow and cleanse and landslide: I am the elements, ready to be born. My universal memory leaves me and I will forget from whence I came.

When my journey on Earth ends, the journey back to

the cell begins, to start anew. A circular life. A perpetual orbiting. Yet always, when I come back to my reality, I find myself with a problem: living.

Do the cosmos, my family, everyday politics, nature influence, change, or rule my life? Are we all a part of a gigantic, synchronic clock? Can I do without the clock? Can the clock do without me?

How do I confront my problem?

As I sit and ponder these questions, I take out paper and pencil and begin to draw a diagram. First I draw a circle representing the orbiting universe. Inside this circle I draw a square, each side symbolizing the four traditional elements: earth, water, fire, and air. Inside the square I draw a big triangle signifying the family, society, and government. Inside this triangle I draw a smaller one, formed by the body, intellect, and emotions. Then I think, if I return to the beginning of my journey, outside the universe, I will have to penetrate the circle, the square, the big triangle, and ultimately, the small triangle, where I will dwell. In the process of coming to my destination, I will become imbued with all of them. I can live in the small triangle, but I am all over the diagram. I have a feeling of belonging. I know that I am not alone because when my death comes the diagram will remain, and someone else will take over what I will leave behind.

Once I accept my place on earth, I question where I am going. If I use my imagination, I can go wherever I please and I can experience the only freedom I will ever know. However, I also view my world pragmatically, because I want to know my limitations about going, becoming, owning, and being owned. I try to learn as much as I can about the circle, the square, and the triangles. I am certain I must meet the world's demands, but I would like to make sure that the world will meet mine as well. In the process of orbiting, we all have duties and rights to fulfill.

How do I tell you about family, society, and government? How do I shake you up, show you how they shape and control our lives?

We are not living on an island, and, if we were, we still would have the need to talk, love, and care for someone. We need a structured habitat so we can be cared for if we are ill, or provided for if we are unable to work. We need a language in order to communicate, a heritage to remember and be proud of, and a share of this gigantic planet—a place where we will be welcomed upon our arrival.

Don't we all have a family, a society, a government to talk about? Or should we feel, as in the title of the book by the Peruvian writer Ciro Alegria, that *Broad and Alien Is the World*? For many, it is. This negative, though realistic, attitude is a terrible way to live.

I refuse to be another immigrant on this planet. This is my Earth! Nonetheless, how many times do we feel we don't belong here? That we were born in the wrong world? I will not accept this feeling. I want to walk inside the big triangle and live within it, my identity intact. I refuse to be another number.

I read history and I see people creating methods to enslave people. I feel centuries of war reflected in our calendars. From childhood on, we are trained to be obedient, dependent beings, to fulfill a stereotyped role in our social environment. We are criticized for our lack of good qualities far more often than we are praised for our virtues and our achievements. We live our lives surrounded by hunters. We may even feel that we are here to be tamed, controlled, disposed of. Not only is the world broad and alien, but sometimes I feel that my house, my office, my street no longer belong to me.

When I shave tomorrow morning whom shall I meet in the mirror? Waiting outside the door of my inner life is the world within the big triangle of family, society, and government. I know that sooner or later I will have to open that door and face my external reality. If we find a meaning for ourselves, for our presence, for our permanence on earth, life will also have a meaning. Only then will the pain of being alive ease and only then will we be able to emerge within a world that belongs to us.

The main goal in life is to become free. To achieve freedom we need knowledge and health. Knowledge, health, and freedom compose the foundation on which an integral being stands.

To go through the process of changing for the better we should not expect swift changes because those are the changes that do not last. Magic will not do the job for us. We have to do it ourselves. We should read, listen, observe, and, most of all, question. Learning to become and remain an integral being is predicated on endless questioning.

To undertake our mission we have to position ourselves in truth and the right understanding. To position ourselves in lies and wrong understanding means we will become lost. To be lost in a city is never as frightening as being lost within ourselves. To become an integral being requires effort, every day of our lives. Every day is sacred, and we should perform the ceremony of living as a sacred rite.

There are some disadvantages to becoming an integral being. Much sacrifice is required. If we become stronger and healthy, independent and self-reliant, we may provoke embarrassment, envy, and even anger in those who wish to maintain the status quo. Old relationships may break off, and new ones may be established. These disadvantages must be considered before you begin your search for integration.

This is not a self-help book, but a book geared to the transformation of self by challenging the self's present status. I wrote this book to share my ideas of what each of us should do to live a full life with health, dignity, and independence.

At times in this book I will raise a question, and I will give an answer. But other times perhaps a question will go unanswered, and you will have to ask me one. In any case, I will always offer the seed of a thought you can sow in your own world.

The goal of becoming an integral being must be fulfilled here and now because our reality is here and now. I want you to change today and not tomorrow. Tomorrow is hypothetical, a place to put hopes and promises. Today is the challenge, the unavoidable witness of our life.

··· Chapter One

COSMIC INTEGRATION

> A vast similitude interlocks all.
> Walt Whitman, *Leaves of Grass* (1891)

We have to wait for a starry night. Then we will go out, watch the sky, and let the silence pervade our senses. We should remain still, because we will be overwhelmed by the vastness of a universe that watches us as we watch it.

What do we share in common with the universe?

Had Earth remained covered by one big cloud, as Venus still is, we would never have known of the existence of other planets and stars. Had we, as humans, remained covered by a cloud—our mother's womb—we would never have known of the natural world around us. Fortunately, we have learned that things move: Earth moves around the sun; we move through land, sea, and air; and red cells move through the veins and vessels inside our bodies.

We are all particles of light, energy, and movement. Most important, we are part of the cosmos, and we all interact.

When we lie on a beach on a sunny day, we will burn in a couple of hours, yet the sun is 93 million miles away. But for our skin, how near it is!

A sunny day makes us feel good, a cloudy day, gloomy. The presence or absence of sunlight determines the shades of colors, which affect our emotions. For years we have known that people living closer to the equator appear to be happier, a fact reflected in their social behavior and music. Those living closer to the Arctic or Antarctic are prone to depression, social withdrawal, and drinking to forget rather than to celebrate. Recent research indicates that sunlight, real or artificial, can relieve depression in certain individuals. The results are as satisfactory as those obtained with antidepressant medications.

The moon also affects us. It has been worshipped in our religions, it has challenged our scientific minds, and it has seduced our poets. In this century, it has accepted our astronauts on its surface. The strong connection between the moon and humanity is evident in a woman's menstrual cycle, which lasts 28.5 days, the same length as the lunar cycle. Folk tales, popular and scientific knowledge confirm the relationship of the moon to behavior. In medieval times, mental patients were called *lunatics*, derived from the Latin word for moon, *luna*. Scientific investigations point toward a relationship between behavior and lunar periodicity. Emotional disorders, particularly aggression, have been observed to worsen during a full moon.

Another influence is gravitation, a force that produces attraction among planets and keeps us bound to earth. Consequently, we cannot fly like birds, a fact I resent in the spring.

Gravitation also affects our biology. The 1976 studies of Dr. F. A. Brown explain some of the mysteries of biological rhythms. In an experiment, oysters were shipped from the Connecticut shore to Dr. Brown's laboratory in Evanston, Illinois. There the oysters continued to open their shells to correspond with the time of the high tides in Connecticut. The oysters were responding to biological rhythms. After two weeks, however, the oysters began to open their shells when the moon would have caused high tides had Evanston been a coastal city. In other words, they opened their shells when the moon was at its zenith over their new home in Illinois.

Dr. Brown's experiment is but one example of the perfect balance within nature, a balance that is reflected across the universe. Part of this balance is maintained by electromagnetic forces keeping things together—for instance, atoms. Without these forces, we would break down into small particles.

Almost every organism, including humans, is ruled by biological clocks related to the patterns of day and night, known as circadian rhythm. This approximately twenty-four-hour cycle modifies hormonal secretion, temperature, sleep, and blood levels of certain substances. The circadian cycle can be disturbed by traveling against the clock, causing what is called the jet lag syndrome, a disruption in bodily functions. For this reason, athletes, for instance, fly to their sites of competition ahead of time in order to normalize their circadian rhythms before they perform.

The ancient Egyptians first observed a relationship between weather conditions and health. In Greece, both Hippocrates and Aristotle pointed out the influence of weather on disease. Heat, humidity, cold, and barometric pressure affect the functions of the body.

For hundreds of years, popular beliefs as well as empirical observations by physicians assigned the cause of certain changes in our physiology (for example, lethargy, instability) to winds. The hot, dry versions such as the Pampero (Argentina), the Sirocco (Italy), the Mistral (France), the Foehn (Germany), the Sharav (Israel), the Santa Ana (Southern California), and the winds of the Sahara are some of the culprits said to produce physical changes. In 1973, Dr. F. G. Sulman, of the Hebrew University of Jerusalem, reported exhaustion of the adrenal glands and overproduction of other hormones of the body during the hot, dry, windy season of the Sharav. Migraines, blood clotting, and bone pains are also influenced by weather changes.

We are all connected to the universe in which we live and to its four elements. By breathing, we are connected to air; by drinking, to water; by eating, to animals, plants, and minerals, and the soil; by the need for heat and our own heat, to fire.

Fire is a very old element on earth, which can probably be traced back to lightning. The Beijing man was able to use fire a half million years B.C. However, the Beijing man didn't know that we are also fire because we produce heat, that we can burn like a log, that we are combustible. Self-combustion has been reported at different times in many parts of the world. This phenomenon takes place suddenly, and reduces the person to ashes. No external or internal forces capable of causing it have been found, and it remains a mystery yet to be solved.

Why do we need to know about the relationship between ourselves and nature? Each time we forget, or try to forget, nature, it is at our peril. Earthquakes demolish what we build, floods wash away houses and livestock, hurricanes sweep away our technology, droughts wither our crops. Nature constantly reminds us of our place on earth. How can we pollute the water, contaminate the atmosphere, defoliate the jungles, make the air radioactive, and still pretend that we are the kings of creation?

We have grown away from nature because part of our destiny is to invent, create, and discover. But human folly often takes over, replacing functions performed by nature and by ourselves. We have developed a highly technological world in which our latest aim is to replace human intelligence with computers. But what will happen to our rusty brains?

We cannot be replaced. An artificial world of technology cannot think, love, or get angry for us. We may use our knowledge, but we should never abuse it. Anything that goes against nature is eventually destroyed by it. Therefore, if we persist in believing that we are not part of nature, but its masters, we will be lost. The proof is all around us. We are already overwhelmed by a technology turning against us. Many of us live ridden by despair, boredom, and loneliness.

Yet we are part of nature—at least when we walk along the seashore, or when we immerse ourselves in a forest, smell the leaves, the flowers, the air after a rain. We enjoy the water we drink, our thoughts, the people we love. We respond to an animal or to a plant. We need to touch nature with our hands. We need to get wet in the rain, experience cold in the winter, and sweat in the summer in tune with circadian rhythms, so our senses will be fed, and our bodies and intellect will find harmony with nature.

We must search for our place in nature, in the cosmos, and know who we are, for ourselves and for others. To do this, we have to find ourselves: learn to know our inner desires, inclinations, defects, virtues. We have to accept ourselves as we are, and change what we dislike about ourselves. We must love ourselves in order to endure and to enjoy life as much as we can.

Who am I for others?
Who am I for myself?

We can be many beings, play many roles. For a parent, one can be a son; for a sibling, a brother; for the government, a citizen; for a politician, a voter; for the military, a soldier; for the police, a perpetrator or a victim. When asked, "Who are you for the universe?" the Spanish thinker and writer Miguel de Unamuno answered, "For the universe, I am nothing, but for me, I am everything."

Unamuno was right. Since I was a little boy I sensed my aloneness—even when surrounded by people. The aloneness of New York City, of a big railroad station at rush hour. When I was sixteen I wanted to be told that I existed. The Cartesian principle, "I think, therefore I am," was not enough. I wanted someone else's confirmation of my presence on this earth. I wanted to be deeply loved. I could not accept the idea of a routine existence, of a predetermined quota of love and pain. Passion, intensity of life were important elements to make living worthwhile. I did not want to be a cipher neatly fitting into a statistical column.

Every morning I used to applaud myself in front of a mirror, saying out loud how great I was—a rudimentary way of curing my shyness. But who was I? Was I my skin covered with acne? Was I the orphan who overheard people expressing pity? Was I the soldier who was told, "You serve your country by polishing the boots of your officers"? Was I the medical student who was not allowed to challenge the teaching of the great professors?

I am, as Buddha said hundreds of years ago, forces, movements. I am a dynamic concept, a continuous oscillation from light to energy, and vice versa, the basic concept of quantum philosophy. Nonetheless, I am Anibal Yaryura-Tobias, trying to equate the vastness of the life force with the commonplace act of having to pay a monthly electric bill.

Yes, Unamuno was indeed right. If we are nothing for the universe in which we live, we had better do something about ourselves; otherwise, we will perish. If we care about others, we won't be able to give what we don't have. If we want to share we must first have; only then will we be able to help others.

On a small scale, however, we are also a universe. Like the universe, we are not completely explored. Within ourselves remain regions unknown to our senses. The final chapter of our anatomy, emotions, and intellect has yet to be written. Our connection with the universe is slowly being explained by physics, chemistry, higher levels of consciousness, and the long-term experience of living on this planet. Rutherford, Planck, and Einstein were three physicists whose findings have opened the door to an era of revolutionary knowledge still not appreciated in its extraordinary dimensions.

Ernest Rutherford showed us that atoms consist of vast regions of space in which small particles move. These subatomic units of matter can be present either as particles or as waves. This duality is also present in light, which can take the form of an electromagnetic wave or a particle. Max Planck discovered that the energy of heat radiation is emitted intermittently, in the form of "energy packets." Albert Einstein advanced the theory that light can also appear in the form of energy packets, or "quanta," now called "photons." These particles have no mass and travel with the speed of light.

The ability of energy to become light, and vice versa, may be useful in filling gaps that exist in our relation to the universe. It is a physical phenomenon that shows the fluctuation between reality and the process of becoming reality. It could also help to prove the physical existence of the beyond or the spiritual world. Perhaps the existence of soul, in its religious sense, could be explained in terms of physics. The soul may physically exist as a particle, a wave, or a light. After our death it could leave our body as a wave and travel far away. Similar conclusions have been arrived at in Hinduism, which describes the soul as a beam of light. Fritjof Capra, in his book *The Tao of Physics,* attempted to show the parallel between physics and Eastern mysticism.

Undoubtedly, there is a cosmic interconnectedness still in the process of being discovered that relates to each of us. This cosmic network is similar to our brain, which is also a web of atoms and subparticles. In a way, the cosmos is a thinking brain, and our brain a thinking cosmos. Our imagination continuously creates personal "universes." Whether these ever materialize cannot be either proved or disproved, but we certainly know that whoever created the universe had to first "think" of it.

Unfortunately, we are too busy with our daily routines to explore life beyond the scope of our physical senses. That is why it is important to wake the dormant regions of our brain so we can develop our senses to the fullest and reach frontiers beyond our current comprehension. Only then will we wed the cosmos.

We must become wild horses and roam prairies and valleys, become condors and dream at the summits of mountains. By galloping and flying we may absorb freedom in its totality of vast isolation and silence. But we are still light, the wetness of dawn, and the space that explodes on the horizon or contracts when lips become kisses. Poetry or chemistry, wild dreams or rigid laws, mysteries of ancient civilizations, the hidden objects of what we call "nothingness," all are reflected in ourselves: magnificent creatures carrying an unexploited load of love, curiosity, and creativity. We are chaos in the process of becoming an integral being. It was Nietzsche who said that from chaos a star may be born.

We must narrow the gap between knowledge and ignorance. Our educational system, whether implemented at home or at school, lacks freedom, imagination, and practicality. We are offered educational material that confines our thinking to preestablished facts. And we have been wrong. It was believed that energy could not be liberated. Today we have nuclear power. Consider building a television or submarine a thousand years ago. We thought we could never fly. Outer space is now old news. All of these ideas were considered nonsensical, to put it mildly, in the past. Fortunately, rebellious, creative brains challenged the status quo and proved otherwise.

It is the work of a very few people that keeps the world growing spiritually, scientifically, and technologically. Must we forever be followers? There is a world out there that is invisible, untouchable, soundless, tasteless, and odorless. We either call that world the beyond, or else we flatly deny its existence. Knowledge, meditation, and intellectual flexibility will unfold the evidence to bring the universe together as a single entity. The words *mystery, secret,* and *occult* will be erased from our vocabulary. Reality will emerge as a unifying force. The quality of life will improve because it will have meaning, where before it was rife with absurdity.

To reach our goals, we are given an allotted time on earth—roughly seventy years. If we have been here as humans for one million years, and if we understand how little one million years is in the context of the universe, imagine how minute a duration of seventy years is for us, the individual, on earth.

We have now introduced ourselves to the concept of time.

We are born and we will die; a star is born and it will die. Even the ocean dies a little when it evaporates. Life and death follow each other; we learn that we are not eternal, except in our hope to achieve eternity. To a butterfly, the life of a tortoise may seem an eternity. It is all a matter of how we perceive time.

We may conceive of time as an illusion of the mind or an invention that brings order to our daily lives.

Some researchers, such as Jean Charon, have wondered whether space contracts itself around a vehicle. If this theory is correct, we could travel, in a vehicle, great distances within a lifetime, because the distance would shrink.

As a particle, time moves forward and backward. In other words, past and future disappear. When light leaves a star to reach Earth, for instance, nothing can be done to intercept its arrival. A beam of light traveling toward Earth is already the star's past and the future on Earth. Yet it is the same light beam, traveling at such speed and over such distances, that renders our concept of time senseless.

We will feel more comfortable if we consider time as our process of becoming, like growing, or like movement. Time does not stop. Even if we remain in the dark, without external stimuli, we will experience the passage of time in our mind. There is no cessation of time in this universe, except in death.

Death reminds us of the presence of time: an ongoing phenomenon—our life—ends. Therefore, the termination of anything, whether it is a plant, a season, or a creature, indicates the existence of time. Yet we in our stubbornness refuse to accept the idea of our mortality. Most of us believe that everyone will die but us. However, because immortality is a figment of our imagination, philosophical devices have been provided to palliate our departure. The Persian religious reformer Zoroaster (628 to 551 B.C.) preached the idea of a final judgment in which the dead would be resurrected. This belief was to be shared by Pharaonic Egypt, Jews, Christians, and Muslims, and by Buddhism, with its belief in recurrent birth or reincarnation.

We are all concerned with time; we are enslaved and diseased by it. Either we don't have enough of it or it never seems to pass.

The precision of atomic clocks has shown that due to a slowing down of the earth's rotation, we add an extra second per year to our annual time. This may not upset our present or future plans, but it clearly indicates our interest and attachment to time and, subsequently, to eternity.

We live in a circular pattern of existence, from birth to death, and we learn that in order to live our allotted time, we have to interact with other objects that share the universe with us: animals, plants, oceans, moons, and stars.

In Ecclesiastes, it is said that there is a season for everything, a time for every purpose under heaven; a time to be born and a time to die, a time to plant and a time to reap.

Time recording, or chronobiology, has not always been accepted in the same way throughout history. Time cycles, eras, and epochs were recorded in terms of geographical or cosmic changes, or major historical events. The most widely accepted method of time counting is the Christian calendar, worked out by Dionysius Exiguus of Rome in the sixth century. It took five hundred years to agree upon the date of Christ's birth and to make that year zero. Why did Western civilization wipe out a few million preceding years? Every time we write a letter now, we notate only a couple of thousand years of history.

Perhaps in our aim to conquer eternity, we have chosen to shrink an important factor: the aging of the world. And it is part of our human nature—don't we often shrink our age? Meanwhile, we face the time span of our individual lives. I experience my own time as an actual melting process with a candle lighted by my parents when they gave birth to me—a candle that I blow out every birthday, until the day it will melt away forever.

Time is the worst slave master I have ever encountered. The ideal is to live a continuous present that takes us from point A, our birth, to point B, our death. Life is an exhibition along the road. We have the freedom to walk in and out of its various concessions as we please. We can sit and rest or keep on walking. Those who walk behind us live their present in our past, those who walk ahead of us live their present in our future.

Louis Pauwels and Jacques Bergier said, in *Le Matin des magiciens*, "Freedom is being able to be, inside eternity that already is." How can we become ourselves inside eternity? The best way would be by blending ourselves with time, energy, and matter, by accepting our temporary presence on earth as a necessary stopover on our way to becoming eternity. To accomplish this would be to achieve the integral state of being. To fuse with the totality of the universe.

How do we go about becoming an integral being?

Essentially, by being healthy in body, soul, and mind, by being in balance with our environment. We have to learn how to keep ourselves in good mental, emotional, and physical shape and learn how to harmonize with the world. Universal equilibrium can be reached by integration and knowledge. Both will give us the patience to accept things as they are, the will to change what is unfit, and the hope to persevere through sacrifice and discipline.

Therefore, let us cover the basic knowledge that will allow us to put ourselves on the path to improve our lives in an integral manner. By doing so we will develop an orderly self, in harmony with the cosmos.

••• Chapter Two

THE FAMILY

> The Family! Home of all social evils, a charitable institution for indolent women, a prison workshop for the slaving breadwinner, and a hell for children.
>
> August Strindberg, *The Son of a Servant* (1886)

The textbook definition of the family describes it as a union of a man and a woman for the purpose of physical and emotional security, and sexual gratification. From this union, children may be born and the race perpetuated. In ancient Rome, "family" described the group of household servants, or the household head and all those related to him by birth or marriage. It is curious that what we understand about the word *family* now was once linked to the word *servant*. Was family once a place for slavery, rather than love, growth, and fulfillment? Are we still slaves to our families? For those who wish to be free, it is an important question.

The family is the natural arena to develop the integral being. Being born into the wrong family can wreak havoc with someone trying to become an integral being.

In primitive times, families were known as tribes and were run by patriarchs who owned cattle, farms, or land. Families performed many tasks together, such as hunting, farming, and raising children. Originally, families were formed through incestuous relations, which were then socially accepted to fulfill biological needs. But in order to halt the effects of inbreeding, families began to marry into other social groups. These new families began to live under the same roof, and several generations, known as extended families, lived in the same household.

The biological and geographical expansion of families was the origin of society. The family is the germinal unit of society, and family and society complement each other. Through thousands of years the family structure has undergone drastic changes, from patriarchal polygamic systems to the current monogamic quasi-egalitarian construct.

Albeit brief, this review of the origin of the family should stimulate you to become acquainted with the history of your own family. How many know the names of your great-grandparents? The age of your parents? Knowledge of our roots gives us a sense of belonging in time.

We marry to obtain social recognition as an established union and to protect the economic gains obtained throughout the duration of the marital contract. We also marry because our culture has taught us to marry. When people are asked why they marry, they give one or more reasons: "My parents did," "It is socially expected," "To have children," "What will I do when I am old and alone?" "For sex," "Lower taxes." Less pragmatic, and more romantic, are other answers: "Because I'm in love," "To share my life with someone," "To become one in another one."

To become integral beings, we should marry independent of social and religious norms. The decision to marry should be left to our own judgment and to the interplay of our passions and feelings of belonging toward our beloved. Nowadays, marriage can easily be damaged by those unaware of its value.

We live in a society of different cultural prejudices, beliefs, and values. Therefore we tend to wed within our own social, ethnic, and economic circles. Intellectual compatibility, cultural values, religious beliefs, and a similar philosophy of life also play a role. Only a very special breed of people, ready to endure the ostracism imposed by family and society, can make a religious, racial, or economic intermarriage succeed. An integral man and woman, however, will be able to intermarry successfully, because they will know how to handle the societal pressures that can break up a marriage.

It has been said that we marry families rather than individuals. Most of us have not received training in how to get married, but we come from family constellations where people are or were married, and those role models are what we consciously, or unconsciously, use as learning material. Our desire to wed is part of the learning process reflecting our family's behavior. How important it is to be born to integral parents! To watch them perform the ceremonial acts of love, care, respect, and tolerance. It is from them that we learn to hug and kiss, to hold hands, and to share the time of togetherness. We should be grateful if we see our parents telling each other, "I love you." Some of us live in angry homes where the word *love* is never spoken. And some of us come from broken homes. If we do come from a home like that, what can we do? We must look for examples elsewhere, we must follow the good marriages of others—the parents of a close friend, or married neighbors. Living with a stepparent whose marriage is good may change our negative feelings about marriage.

One should marry only when there is a solid foundation

of love, a will to carry on a long lasting commitment, a mutual companionship, a desire to share lives, and agreement on feelings about having children. When we are pronounced husband and wife, we exchange rings. The ring, as a symbol, is a magic circle. It has been worn as a sign of authority, as a bond between a king and his people, as the alliance of church and God, and as an honor. A wedding ring is presented as a symbol of material unity and fidelity. However, if we think that by using a magical object like a ring we will remain faithful and married, we are headed for trouble.

As a worker in mental health I have isolated seven essentials to prevent a marriage from failing: mutual respect, love, trust, sharing, division of work, loyalty, and dialogue. I list mutual respect first, for without respect, no human relationship can survive.

Marriage does not give us ownership of our spouse. If we want service, we should pay for it. The idea of "I am the breadwinner, you wait on me when I come home" is a false one. Both spouses are working people—whether working on the outside or inside of the house. Household work is work. Raising children is very hard work. Therefore, the concept of sharing and division of work is not only fair but essential. We should not marry to compete with or to envy our spouse's achievements. In today's society, where some women have become the main breadwinners, rivalry and resentment are expected. Many husbands find this role reversal difficult to handle. Aggression, depression, and infidelity are some of the mechanisms utilized by husbands to protect their damaged virility. If one is presented with this situation, an honest and open discussion may prevent the deterioration of the marriage. Marriage should be neither a battleground nor a factory for disagreements.

But economic problems, boredom, severe stress, children as the priority, sexual dissatisfaction, taking family life too seriously, and lack of romance may be reasons for discord.

One way to solve economic problems is to determine a household budget, avoiding consumerism and trying to keep up with the Joneses.

Boredom can easily occur in homes where routine activities and a task-oriented life-style are the rule, in couples who are fearful, and thus unable to take risks or embark on adventure. The cycle of coffee, the morning paper, a nine-to-five job, the six o'clock news, dinner, dishes, and bed is hardly inspirational.

Severe stress, one price of modern society, is usually indicated by irritability, low tolerance, loss of sexual desire, and mental and physical fatigue. Stress and its symptoms are a time bomb that can blow apart the family constellation.

Some marriages are threatened when children are placed ahead of all else. Children must not take precedence over the needs of the couple. Roles as spouses and parents should be well defined, with boundaries established. Husbands and wives require as much care as children because eventually the children will leave, and they will be left behind.

For most people, sex is the ruler by which to measure how a marriage is doing. Sexual problems usually reflect an underlying marital conflict. Yet sex is hardly the primary reason for divorce. Although important, it is not the only key to a successful marriage. In a culture such as ours, ridden with guilt about sex, marriage makes sex socially acceptable. However, even married couples may feel guilty about having sex, because they lack sufficient knowledge about it, or because sex seems sinful, immoral, or burdensome to them. In some ancient Middle Eastern cultures women were taught that their prospective husbands would "bother" them, meaning they would expect sexual intercourse. In today's modern society, many women and men also feel "bothered" by having to fulfill their marital "duties." Consequently, they either deny the problem or choose other outlets.

Couples must have a sense of humor about their family life. Taking family life too seriously will create an air of impending doom, depression, worry, and frustration within the walls of a house. Sometimes family life can be as entertaining as any situation comedy on television. We can be funny; we are funny. It depends on how we react to daily events. Rigidity of attitude and inflexibility of judgment can complicate a marriage and family life.

For a marriage to work, the art of flirting must be continually practiced. The idea that husbands passively accept wives with curlers, and wives accept potbellied husbands should be obliterated. Every day should be a love affair and every night a wedding night.

Family life must by definition be creative. The monotony of the day should be challenged. We should prepare a weekly schedule of changing activities, from the preparation of a new dish to the rearrangement of furniture. A house's colors, textures, pictures, walls, and even plants should reflect the personalities of its dwellers. The house, our most private territory, should blend with nature as well.

When married couples are asked whether they have children, if the answer is yes, they will never be asked why. But should the answer be no, a surprised "Why not?" will follow. I feel more inclined to ask why we have children, because having children entails responsibilities many people may not be able to assume. When I think of these duties—love, care, teaching, guidance, and years of economic support—I question how people who don't love themselves, or who are self-centered or hardly able to make ends meet, manage to be parents.

People who are not interested in having children should not feel bound by society to have them. There are many reasons why people choose not to have children. They may want the freedom to pursue careers. They may believe that children impose obligations they will not be able to fulfill. There are individuals who feel incapable of assuming a parental role. Because they are responsible people, they choose to behave responsibly and not have children.

Too many people have children because of a need to prolong themselves on this earth, or because of social or religious pressure. To be a parent is a matter of vocation. If we don't have the vocation for parenthood, we will do a poor job as parents, and, as a result, the family will become diseased.

Social and religious groups may have a vested interest in our children. In the recent past, child labor was common practice in many societies. The exploitation of children by industrial and farming societies has not disappeared and, in fact, is growing. Religious institutions count on increasing the number of their believers not only through preaching and conversions, but through reproduction among their members.

When the first child is born we rush to buy Dr. Spock's book. We are surrounded by veteran parents, including our own, and by the pediatrician. We would love to see our children become what we could not and excel in areas where we failed. The best heritage we can offer them is an education and our best model: a life of integrity.

Raising children is an art because it requires intuition, creativity, and a dash of borrowed experience. The task should be carried out by both parents, mother and father, who must reach an understanding about how they are going to raise their children. Unfortunately parents, having their own theories, often fail to agree upon how their children should be raised. Although the Bible says that God created man in his image and likeness, we should not raise our children in our own image and likeness. We should bring them up as integral beings, guiding our children's growth within the framework of health, freedom, and mutual respect, in harmony with the world.

Once we have decided upon a set of rules to raise our children by, these rules should be firmly implemented. Firmness is very important, because children need not only security, but certainty. A "yes" always has to mean yes, and a "no" always has to mean no. It is useful for the emotional state of our children to explain our behavior. An affirmative or negative response should always be preceded by an explanation. Children will be grateful because we are showing them not only love and care, but respect.

As parents we must judge, praise, reward, punish, approve, and disapprove. However, home should not become a courthouse. A Jesuit maxim says: "Give me a child for the first six years of life and he'll be a servant of God till his last breath." A child is not a slave but a free person, an individual who will often surprise us with a need for risk and adventure. We should allow our children to be free, otherwise we will be taking away their natural identities. We should allow our children to follow their vocation, permitting them to be whatever they want to be. We are unique, and so are our children.

The following letter describes the incipient presence of an integral being who, at the age of four, is already defending her individuality.

Dear Anibal,

As you requested, the following is pretty much a verbatim account of Danielle's disagreement with me when I told her that I had made an appointment for her to get a haircut:

Danielle: "Why did you make an appointment for a haircut for me? You didn't even ask me first. You had no right. I don't want a haircut. I'm going to let it grow long. You wear your hair like you want it, and I wear my hair like I want it, and I could have my hair however I want it to be. My hair is none of your business. It's part of my body so it is my business."

After she had the haircut she had agreed to only for a trim, but I had quietly suggested to the hairdresser that she make it a "short trim," Danielle expressed her disappointment and anger with a quiet and resigned tone: "I told you that I only wanted a trim but I guess you didn't hear me."

Best regards,
Emily

At one point in our childhood, all of us would like to emulate our heroes—a nurse, a firefighter, an astronaut—but aren't our parents our first heroes? Parents are powerful beings, invested with divine qualities. We love and fear them as we love and fear our gods. Parents care, love, and provide for us, but they can also punish or abandon us. We debate our dependency toward them and our continuous need for their approval, regardless of how old we are. In our imagination, we may kill our parents, but later we bring them back to life. We keep explaining, excusing, condoning, and forgiving our parents and their presence stays with us forever.

The worst thing that can happen to a parent is for one to lose his or her aura of deity. To face their children off guard—weak, unwise, doubtful, or fearful—signals a new stage of the parent-child relationship. The parent's transition from an almighty figure to an average individual occurs during the child's puberty. The experience should be accepted with joy because it announces the passage of childhood into adolescence. Children should be reassured during this time of the continuous presence of parents, and that they are active participants in family life.

To organize a family as we desire requires adequate planning and division of power. Decision making has been traditionally delegated to the father in patriarchal systems and to the mother in matriarchates. The active participation of women as wage earners in the so-called man's world has taken away man's supremacy as head of the household. In well-structured families, decision making also takes into consideration the opinions of the children. Having children contribute to planning the daily activities of the house and making them aware of the economic difficulties or the emotional problems faced by the family gives them a sense of belonging and respect. Finally, it teaches them how to run their own families in years to come.

Our concept of family changes with our growth. The way we see our family when we are children is not the way we will perceive it when we become adults. Family means different things for different people. For me, family was my grandfather presiding at the dining room table, surrounded by his wife and fifteen children. His idea of family may be overwhelming by present standards; for me, it was an experience that helped make me the way I am today. It is an unforgettable memory of love and togetherness.

Our family can make or destroy us. If we face excessive emotional disappointment in our family life, we should question what is lacking. Is it love? Is it an inability to share? Is it a resistance to work as a family group? Is it economic hardship?

As in a marriage, respect, love, trust, dialogue, and sharing are required to keep a strong family bond. It is important to let other members of the family know that we love them. We ought to verbalize it. Say, "I love you." Let us show grudges as well. It's important to share with the family what we have and who we are. Sharing what we have is relatively easy, but it is becoming more difficult to share who we are. We are moving inward, becoming self-centered. Isolating the self is not a characteristic but a consequence of our inability to integrate ourselves with one another.

Praise and approval are very important factors in improving relationships. No matter how old we are, we will ask ourselves, "Would my mother or father approve of it?" Even after our parents' death, we still ask ourselves whether they would approve our behavior, successes, or failures.

Many keep their marriages together because of the children, for economic reasons, for fear of social disapproval, because of religious beliefs, to avoid messy divorces, and for fear of loneliness following the matrimonial break.

How do we keep a marriage intact? Compromise is the rule. If a marriage isn't working, marital counseling is needed. Having the courage to seek help should not cause embarrassment or feelings of failure; on the contrary, it denotes wisdom. Marital therapy may bring into focus the main issues in dispute, issues that become lost amid an overwhelming number of petty incidents.

Although we may not consult anyone before we get married, we must consult and seek advice over and over again in order to avoid a divorce. A divorce is seen as a catastrophe; it is a measure of failure in life. It becomes worse when children are involved. In one of my short stories, I wrote "Marriage is a nocturnal oblivion of what was a diurnal happening; if not it becomes defeated. It is a tragedy to wake up one morning and, instead of getting to know each other again, to remain unknown, then and forever." It is necessary to forgive and heal our quarrels. The decision to divorce is one of life's toughest options.

In the past, when the life span was shorter, the marital cycle was also shorter, and the mutual needs of the couple were less likely to be extinguished. In today's society, a longer life span, linked to a faster life-style, has influenced the duration of a marriage. One year of marriage may equal several years in the past. Some of us reach the conclusion that there is nothing else left to be known after ten, fifteen, or twenty years of marriage. The marital cycle has been completed, the marriage exhausted. We have biological and geophysical cycles, why not emotional and social cycles? Then it may be fair to say that divorce is not the failure of a marriage but its funeral.

Some children are abandoned by their parents, raising fundamental questions for the child. Who were my parents? Why did they give me up? How bad was I for my parents to give me away? Yet how bad can a newborn child be, and why do we blame ourselves for our parents' rejections? Without exception, it is difficult for any of us to admit that our parents were wicked.

How may I become an integral being if my parents gave me away? How do I fill out medical forms when it asks for family history? How will I speak to my children about non-existent grandparents? Do I invent them? I am sad, I cry, I am frightened, and I am angry. I belong to a different breed.

It is a crime to destroy the incipient integral being that is the child. Because children are free, because children question and challenge; they have dreams, they learn quickly, and they are responsible. In a sense, children are almost perfect beings. Not integral. Not yet, for that takes work and learning.

The modern family is confronted with two major social issues: violence within the family and the future of the family.

Violence is reaching epidemic proportions in the family. Because aggressive behavior has permeated every layer of society, the family cannot avoid it. The most common form of aggressive behavior found in the family is verbal attack. Corporal punishment, usually explained as "useful to bringing children up," is also common. Physical assault among spouses is on the increase. Jane O'Reilly reported in *Time* magazine (Sept. 5, 1983) that approximately six million wives are physically abused by their husbands in any one year. Furthermore, some two thousand to four thousand women are beaten to death annually. On the other hand, sociologist Murray Straus has estimated that each year 282,000 men are beaten by their wives. Cases have recently been reported in which children and grandchildren beat their parents and grandparents. The National Center on Child Abuse and Neglect estimates that about 250,000 children are abused annually.

The roots of family violence rarely lie with biological factors, but rather with disturbed personalities. Usually violence is explained in terms of social disease, such as alcoholism or drug addiction. Family violence is present in every socioeconomic class.

Is there anything we can do to prevent or reduce violence? In one study, mothers who were allowed to room with their babies immediately after giving birth were found to be less abusive than mothers who did not see their babies until seven hours after delivery. The researchers concluded that letting mothers assume responsibilities as early as possible may help prevent abuse. Blair Justice, Ph.D., of the University of Texas, says: "Once violence is installed as a way of family life it becomes difficult to reduce it." By the time outside social services move in to investigate the episodes of domestic violence, the family has already been damaged. What remains is to protect the abused member by placing him or her in a foster home, in the case of a child, or in special safe houses, when it comes to wives. Family therapy and intensive individual therapy are also helpful tools in helping to solve the crisis and organize the long-term therapeutic program. In addition, there are specialized agencies that deal with these issues and self-help groups for abused persons. From the social end, a reduction in violence-oriented mass media will undoubtedly benefit violence control.

What is the outlook for the future of the family? Close to the turn of the new century, observe the prototype of the modern family. We see the parents arriving from work and greeting the children, perhaps with a kiss and a hug. They sit in front of the television set and eat a TV dinner. Once in a while, a comment on the program is heard. The ability to converse is virtually lost. Each family member tenaciously holds on to his or her own chair, bedroom, and towel. Family-size deodorants are definitely out. To have guests means extra work. Relatives should remain at a distance. Births, funerals, and weddings are sufficient occasions for seeing each other. This modern family likes being alone. Its members become accustomed to being alone, they withdraw from others, gradually they divorce.

Statistics confirm empirical evidence. According to the U.S. Census Bureau's Population Division, there are 20.6 million single-person homes. The number of single-person homes increased 90 percent from 1970 to 1985. On the other hand, there are now 86.8 million households, of which 72 percent are family units.

Another factor affecting family endurance is family shrinkage. The middle and upper-middle classes are choosing to have smaller families. In addition, some members of the scientific community see overpopulation as a predominant factor in preventing better distribution of food, living space, and wealth. There is growing concern about the danger of overpopulation. Migration to big cities has produced overcrowding and its regrettable consequences: unemployment, poverty, hunger, and violence.

Accordingly, governments fear social unrest due to overpopulation. There has been a noticeable trend to regulate family growth, infringing on the freedom to reproduce. Cases of involuntary sterilization of young girls and women have been reported from various parts of the world. Not all social interference attempts to control growth; many societies ban abortion, and offer sperm banks and test-tube babies. In each case, however, the tight interaction among government, society, and family is continuous.

Today, the family as an institution is threatened. The process of disintegration is visible. Sociologist Carl Zimmerman has put forward a "rise and fall" cyclical theory of family change. Family, as part of history, follows a social pendular system. We have moved from the extended family to the atomistic family, a clear example of social decay. It is up to us to reverse the situation, a situation we can easily repair if we become integral beings.

• • • *Chapter Three*

SOCIETY

> Every social system is more or less against nature, and at every moment nature is at work to reclaim her rights.
>
> Paul Valéry, "The Idea of Dictatorship. Reflection on the World Today" (1931)

Once the human race began to migrate over the earth, geographical borders were established. Social groups remained together to procreate and work, developing a common language, institutions, and traditions. These societies gradually increased their numbers and territories, through natural growth, invasions, wars, and land discoveries. Political organization as nations, unions, federations, and empires resulted.

From their colonies, empires not only obtained raw material for industry, but cheap labor. The economic structure of the Americas could symbolically be represented by a skeleton with the skull of a murdered Indian and the backbone of slaves and immigrant laborers. The Americas, from north to south, blatantly deny their Indian heritage, which was burned and buried so it would be forgotten, and still look to Europe for approval for their fair-skinned biological origin.

Americans, suffused with identity crises, are haunted by

questions: Where do we come from? Who are we? Are we like an adopted child? Are we orphan countries? Young countries, like young people, need an identification.

America is only young from the Caucasian perspective. Otherwise our heritage goes back to 10,000 years B.C. The original inhabitants of the Americas have a profound respect for nature and the universe. Cosmic harmony is not unknown to them. For example, the Andean nation, formed by the Qheswaymara people, organized their societal structure, known as the Tawantinsuyu, in an egalitarian system of distribution of social rights and duties. It is a crime for the community to let someone go hungry. Their history is enriched by a legacy of knowledge in astronomy, agriculture, mathematics, medicine, philosophy, and the arts.

What we have gained in technology, we have lost in the ignorance that made us dismiss the wisdom of our American heritage. A society can be shy, assertive, or aggressive. It can be rich or poor, strong or weak. It can be united by common goals or divided by internal struggle. It may survive on a glorious past, enjoy a prosperous present, or dream of a better future. A society is a portrait of a family, because the foundation of the society is the family. A society integrates itself by accepting different races, creeds, economic and intellectual statuses, but integration is predicated on preserving individual rights.

If a society does not integrate itself—as an integral being does—it will become diseased. Subsequently, each of its members will be affected. Some of them will suffer more than others and may be forced to turn to other societies. It was for that reason that so many people migrated from Europe and Asia to the Americas. People also migrate within their own countries in search of better opportunities. Transience creates socio-emotional imbalance stemming from distrust of newcomers and a need to isolate them from those already integrated into the society. Moreover, immigrants tend to isolate themselves, choosing to dwell where their fellow countrymen have already settled.

Unfortunately, socio-emotional imbalance does not always disappear with time. Our leaders often divide us into artificial social groups, which are far from equal. Leaders tell us about chosen races, religions, and political ideologies. They want us to join them in their beliefs in order to become our social representatives. They compete among themselves for our love and support. Thus we end up being completely divided and alienated from one another, no matter what part of the world we live in.

A segregated society brings uncertainty, fear, oppression, violence, and hatred. The worst discrimination is against the poor and women. With money and power, however, the white will sit with the black, the Jew will marry the gentile, and the atheist will dine with the priest. But acquiring money and power is an unrealistic solution for most of us.

So what do we do? Must we live in a ghetto? As a figure of speech, we all live in intellectual, spiritual, or physical ghettos. Social ostracism, of cultures within cultures, of the wealthy and the poor, of dreamers and pragmatists, surrounds us. The melting pot is a myth. Therefore, we hold on to our assigned ghetto and its traditions—those encompassing the beliefs, practices, food, and folklore of our social group. Traditions give meaning and a sense of belonging to our social self and help us stay in balance with our social environment. Thus, in a nonintegrated society, finding balance within the ghetto is an interim solution.

In countries of mixed heritages, it would benefit their

inhabitants to become acquainted with its existing cultures. We have to know in order to love. To remain ignorant about the ways of life of dominant segments of the population produces further separation of the people.

When I came to the United States, the first thing I did was to read as much as I could: comic books, newspapers, magazines, books on American history, dictionaries on slang, and so forth. The idea was to immerse myself in the evolution of my new country from a formal and popular view. I liked soccer, but I also watched baseball. When my children were born, I became more integrated through them. The acculturation process wasn't easy, but it was rewarding. Today I go about my social life comfortably confident. The worst thing an immigrant can do is to live in the past and force his family to join him.

Neighborhoods are small-scale models of society. The neighborhood is the link between family and society. It is a gathering point for families, the first step we take in finding balance with society. The first tastes of neighborhood are found at the front door, greeting our next-door neighbor, or talking over the fence of our backyard. Coffee klatches, parent-teacher associations, local volunteer groups, community committee affairs, all enlarge our social horizons. We learn the names of our butcher, baker, mail carrier, shoemaker, bank clerk, grocery store owner, and pharmacist. They, in turn, know our names. It is important to know one another. To have our presence acknowledged makes us feel good. In small towns we can still enjoy this familiarity.

Too many societies are allowing communal activities to disappear. In the modern megalopolis with its oversized suburbs, it is often difficult even to find a sidewalk. I can't find enough of them to make a safe trip from my house to my office. Public transportation has been allowed to disintegrate. We travel and commute in isolation in our cars. Main Street, with its shops, is to be found only in memories of the fifties. What counts now are giant shopping mall centers. I am no longer a customer but a shopper with a plastic card that has a forgettable, regrettable number on it. I miss sidewalks on rainy days, the noise of my footsteps on crisp snow, the soda fountain, the ice cream man, my friends on the block, and the policeman on the corner. Who will ever miss the parking lot of a shopping mall?

The loss of identity infuriates me. Often friends and relatives from abroad come to visit. They praise the well-kept gardens of our neighborhood. If it is summer, they will ask why the beautiful yards are empty and why no one is out walking on such a magnificent sunny afternoon. Well, I tell them, perhaps the neighbors are watching television, or shopping, or working extra hours. Who knows?

We are becoming an alienated world in which we are often targets. If we live in cities with a high crime rate, we can be the individual targets of criminals. If we live in a country with a government against its own people, we are the social targets of a dictatorship.

A sense of doom pervades our emotional balance. The concept of a benign world is so fragile that when a physical catastrophe occurs, the length of recovery is long. A social disaster often produces a delayed psychological impact. First we become overwhelmed by the intensity of our emotional reaction. Then we move into a stage of fear and stress. To deny this condition, we may resort to drugs. Others may develop psychosomatic symptoms such as migraines, diarrhea, or insomnia. If the impact is too extreme, we may be unable to function. Then our ability to love, to work, or to cope is lost.

People no longer enjoy their backyards because they are scared. The yard belongs to a hostile world, a diseased social structure, so we stay inside to feel safer. If, in addition, our family is diseased, we will move from the living room to the bedroom. If things get worse we will refuse to get out of bed. A bed is comfortable and warm, and if it comes with a pillow that can be used as a cover for our fears, so much the better. But where do we go from bed?

We have to get up, go out, and fight back. We cannot live without society. We must court, and eventually marry, our society. If society does not accept the marriage, our family becomes isolated and is automatically segregated. Meanwhile, society demands work from our brains and muscles. Our brains will give us all a better world by making discoveries, fighting disease, decreasing poverty, and defeating famine. Our muscles will build houses and roads; we will establish communication and transportation systems.

Nowadays we are able to move around the world and the planets, yet we are far from united. Our brains are used to develop bombs and our muscles to throw them. The destruction of the world and ourselves seems unavoidable.

There are resources that can help us reform the negative impact of society in our lives. There are two primordial conditions needed to maintain a healthy social environment: social cohesion and social control. We need social cohesion, or cultural consensus, on how society dictates the interdependence of its members and, most important, a sense of belonging. We can achieve this by our active participation in social affairs, ranging from town meetings to national politics.

We also need social control and cohesion to live together. As Hobbes said, life without cooperation would be "solitary, poor, nasty, brutish, and short." If we start by exerting self-control, others may do the same. "I don't steal" becomes the equivalent of "You don't steal." If we multiply this behavior, we show cohesiveness on a given moral value. This is an example of social control through cooperation.

But to change our social system for the better permanently, we must educate our young to form a new society—one of freedom and mutual respect. This type of society has to teach children that *they* are the reason for the existence of the social structure. That governments exist only to *protect* their rights to be free, safe, and own property. The principles put forward by Hobbes, Locke, and John Stuart Mill emphasize individual rights over the rights of the state. To preserve these concepts and their application we must work hard for knowledge. Children must be aware from their social start in school why and where they should stand. If schools do not offer a political curriculum, it is up to the parents to educate their children. If parents are uneducated, it is up to our civic organizations to arrange educational campaigns to teach the young discipline, cooperation, and social solidarity.

The availability of freedom varies among today's societies, in which the rights of the state often prevail over the rights of the individuals, yet we all possess essential or vital freedoms. We have the freedom to eat, to sleep, and to work. Then what do I really mean by freedom? I mean the freedom to be what I want to be, to work at what I choose, and to live anywhere in the world. I mean the right to question my government, my society, and my family. I want to be free to fulfill my duties to my fellow beings, uninhibited by social restraints.

We are not as free as we could be. We are putting our

lives in the hands of a few rulers and the prevailing psychosocial norms. Society has conditioned and programmed our lives at its own discretion. We are forced to go to school. To cross a border we must have a permit. From our birth to our burial everything has to be authorized. We are continuously reminded that freedom is a relative right.

Under the present circumstances, we are surrounded by a polluted physical, moral, and intellectual environment in which we are still expected to go about our everyday obligations. We read in the newspaper about the possibility of nuclear war, the creation of a new dictatorship, drought in Africa, babies dying, organized crime and drug traffic, as well as the prevalence of torture, and new ways of importing cheap labor—like the old slave market.

At times my head spins with all this information. A feeling of impotence invades me. What am I to do about it? Just being a psychiatrist and a poet doesn't seem enough. I could decide not to read the papers and go about my business, but when toxic waste is in my water and my basic foods, the job market closes up, a friend is mugged in the street, and a neighbor is raped, I have to question.

We are gullible people. We are told how to cut our hair and what clothes to wear. If we do that, we will be beautiful and successful. Undoubtedly, we want to belong and be accepted, so for that reason we follow social trends. But changing the width of my necktie will not change my personality. Haircuts, fashions, and the like should be individual choices. I refuse to exchange my self-esteem for a brand-name shirt! We are told that it's okay to dress without a tie, that sneakers are fine for your feet, but try getting a job on Wall Street in that attire.

Why are we ready to give up our individuality to conform to social dictates? Are we buying a new belief or a new philosophy of life with a new look? Even when we are on exhibition at the funeral parlor we mask our real selves. We leave as we lived: in disguise.

No one tells us that the making of an individual is dependent on substance, not appearance. Our moral values, our knowledge, our capacity for sacrifice and perseverance are what count. Having that, we have it all.

Society will put us aside if we are poor. Yet we have the right to be poor. A very unwanted right, true. We also have the right to be rich, although in certain countries it is forbidden. It is hard to satisfy governments and societies. We should have the right to work or not to work, as long as we have an honest means to survive. But we are not allowed to be peaceful hobos, exploring the fields or walking beside the railroad tracks. Christ, Mohammad, Indian prophets, and saintly men walked all their lives. Why can't this be acceptable now?

To say at this point in life, "I don't see the meaning of my presence on earth," defeats any attempt to improve our quality of life. Therefore, we must have goals. To be honest, hardworking, and loyal often seems deviant in today's world. Society will accept you only if you have "made it," regardless of the means employed. For most people the means become the end. They spend their entire lives struggling for their means rather than for their goals.

One Sunday night, my wife and I walked down Park Avenue in Manhattan. We were surrounded by silent tall glass buildings carrying the names of international corporations and banks. We encountered an unusual number of people sleeping on benches, in doorways, and on the sidewalks, their belongings in bags. We left the area immediately, uneasy at the thought of being mugged. Today I wonder that perhaps those people instead had been mugged, by the tall buildings with their glass souls.

How can we prevent society from exerting so much power over us?

What can we do to counteract the constant assaults on our health and individual freedom?

The answer, which we must teach our children even as we learn it, is that *we* are society because society is the sum of all of *us*. Therefore, we must assume individual responsibility for the failures of our social system.

In the early seventies, I was the head of the clinical research unit of a federally operated psychiatric hospital in Buenos Aires. One day I was invited to appear on a nationwide television program to present my views on the treatment of institutionalized mental patients. In those years the conditions in state mental hospitals were deplorable. I was acutely and painfully aware of the misery patients had to endure day after day. Psychiatrists were using drugs, electroshock, and straitjackets to excess and resorting to restraining sheets to tie patients to their beds. So I spoke up. On television, I said that the patients would be better off running away.

Needless to say, my job did not last much longer after that. Because of one single statement I threw away all my dreams of teaching, research, and helping needy patients. But I deeply believed I had to take a stand. I left behind suffering, but I also left a message for the mentally ill: If they mistreat you, run away. And there was a good result from my effort. A journalist picked up on the situation and published an exposé.

I am not only a physician for those who require my professional services; I am also a physician for the society in which I live. How can I remain silent when I see so much injustice? All of us have social duties to perform. We have to participate in the process of organizing, supporting, or changing our social structure. In life there are no small people; we are all important, and we can contribute to the development of our social system. Individual contributions begin within our neighborhood, school system, and civic organizations. Voting in local, state, and national elections is essential.

It is important to remember that social awareness is not an inherited quality but one acquired through the process of learning. Life is a challenge that rewards or punishes us with different yardsticks of justice. *Equality* is a word in a dictionary, *justice* an ambiguous term, and *freedom* a scarce commodity. These problems frighten me. But I try to rescue myself from confusion and fear by reading, by acquiring knowledge, by building discipline, and by injecting myself with a capacity for sacrifice and the will to fight back.

We are not alone in the struggle. There are now almost five billion people who are controlled by the social systems in which they live. Individual freedom is possible. The question is, how to get it? Let us read about governments and how they affect our lives and mark our destinies.

••• *Chapter Four*

GOVERNMENT

> Our father who art in heaven
> Stay there. . . .
>
> Jacques Prévert, *Paroles* (1947)

Joe was having his breakfast when the radio broadcaster announced that his country was at war. Ten months later he died in battle.

Jane lived in a country that was economically mismanaged and corrupt. Inflation was rampant, and jobs became scarce. Jane went bankrupt.

Mike was born poor and his family could not feed him properly. He began to show signs of starvation. But a government social agency came to his rescue and provided him with food and medical care. He got well.

Sue could not afford college. But she was born in a country that offered free higher education for all.

Governments have a direct influence on our lives and destinies. Therefore, if we wish to become integral beings, we must know about government. An integral being will not develop within a diseased system.

A government requires power. As we all know, power can be misused and arbitrarily exercised. So the first question is how to limit public power while maintaining a harmonious relationship between government and the citizenry.

The West has formulated political doctrines ranging from the republic of Plato, the pragmatic cynicism of Machiavelli, the utilitarianism of Hobbes, the protection of individual rights of Locke, the "general will" of Rousseau, the anarchism and utopianism of Bakunin, the absolutism of Hegel, and the communism of Marx and Engels. Through the centuries, all of these political systems have been applied in different degrees and modalities. They all claim to improve quality of life and social welfare. But do we need government to improve our lives?

In 1769, Voltaire said, "If God did not exist, He would have to be invented." Why would God have to be invented? To blame someone for the mess in which we live? To be protected and give hope to our desires? As a sensible religious belief to feed our souls? After reading Voltaire I often ask myself whether we would need to create a government if there was none.

We are going through a worldwide crisis in which governments and institutions have fallen short of the expectations of the citizens. Constitutional governments are pseudo-democracies, dictatorships abound, prison systems do not function, hospitals are inadequate, religious institutions focus more on political than on spiritual matters. In some countries there is no right to vote. In others, only one candidate is the contender, and in still others, though people have the right, they choose not to vote. Skepticism and disbelief in government and politicians prevail.

In addition to the central government, we have to deal with "parallel governments" such as multinational corporations, the military, and organized crime, all of which directly or indirectly participate in policy making. Unions, professional societies, and certain religious groups also pressure the state in order to promote their self-interests.

The struggle for power has created an unreliable alliance between government and other seats of power. A fusion of these power systems occurs when important politicians become heads of corporations, or when organized crime has dealings with banks or police departments. All of these alliances have a single aim: the control of people.

Throughout history we have learned of or lived under every conceivable political system, none of which offered an environment of freedom and respect. It is difficult to isolate one single cause for the failure of government and that is why the problem must be approached at different social levels.

A government fails as the result of its own mistakes or because it is established in a diseased society. Because the basic social unit for government is the family, and the family is made up of individuals, the cause of government failure should be investigated in each individual. In general, people are ready to excuse themselves from community or societal responsibilities. If, in addition, the society rejects self-criticism, the government is prone to fail. For a government to function properly, societal endorsement is imperative.

Another cause for government failure is overcentralization. More functions should be delegated to the municipality level. Smaller agencies can be very efficient when given specific tasks. The function of government can also be limited to administration, leaving the ownership of industries, communications, transportation, energy, and so forth to private corporations or cooperatives.

There are concerned citizens who have serious questions about the necessity of government in any form. They believe that government, as it is known, is harmful. Their doctrine, known as anarchism, speaks of a society based on freedom and mutual respect. Their aim is to abolish authority and private property, the sources of social injustice.

Anarchistic ideas were first put forward in the seventeenth century by Gerrard Winstanley, who founded the Digger movement in England, which favored collective farming. In the nineteenth century, French anarchist thought was advanced by Pierre Joseph Proudhon, and in Russia by Mikhail Bakunin and Pyotr Kropotkin. Italian anarchism grew under Enrico Malatesta and German anarchism under Max Stirner. In America, Emma Goldman became a prominent spokesperson for the movement.

At the end of the nineteenth century anarchists were responsible for a series of assassinations and terrorist acts. These activities clearly contradicted anarchism's ideas of freedom and mutual respect and led to the movement's decline. Still, I view anarchism as an ideology of evolution rather than revolution. Mutual respect without authoritarian figures dictating our fates should not be looked upon as a utopian desire but as a feasible goal by which we can attain a higher level of consciousness and morality.

In *Metamorphoses,* Ovid described a golden age without laws in which freedom and beliefs were respected as long as people behaved well toward others. Perhaps one day this type of society will exist and peace will prevail. Meanwhile, we must deal with the reality of government today.

Sociologist Howard S. Becker described a hierarchy of credibility in the social structure. Those at the top of the institution have "the right to define the way things really are." This is similar to the family hierarchy: a child admires the father or mother as a superior physical and mental being because the child does not know any better. Likewise, the less the people of a country know, the more credulous they become about those who head their country. In order to rule, the government must control. This control is exerted through reasoning and power. Control is inherent in human nature. We want to control our futures and the outcome of history. Unfortunately, we also attempt to control each other, and for that reason we enslave, segregate, incarcerate, and kill, which endangers the existence of the integral being. The integral being wants to be free. If a government forces us into a war, or dictates our right to get married or divorced, or to be gay or straight, that government threatens the survival of the integral being.

To avoid excesses of authority we use laws to regulate the use of public power. Laws are sets of rules or regulations that help governments and societies live in harmony. To accept a law we must know the sources of its authority, its application in society, and its moral value. For the integral being, the evaluation and criticism of law are essential, because laws bind us to a life-style. Every human being develops a sense of moral law by which we are able to reason and distinguish good from evil and socialize without harming others. Nonetheless, with so many people in the world with different customs and mores, laws vary. Islamic, Chinese, Hebrew, and Western common law are examples of laws designed to serve social groups with differing philosophies of life.

The law has to be not only just but dynamic. Just because it should conform to the need for equality, and dynamic because norms and attitudes fluctuate through the years. A law may not fit our individual needs. Then the majority rules. A law may infringe upon our moral values. For instance, a religious person may object to war and refuse to go. Do we have the moral right not to obey the law? Or do we try to change the law to consider religious objectors?

There are laws that benefit vested interests to the detriment of the community. For example, zoning laws that allow more high-rise buildings in already overcrowded, dark cities, tax laws that favor huge corporations, and so on. What can we do to correct unfair laws? We can work through our community organizations, civic groups, or neighborhood boards for change, and we can vote.

Together with the law, mass media is another important link between a government and its subjects as it sends information, back and forth. This two-way flow should be honest and complete. Partial reporting or suppression of news can lead to misinformation or disinformation, so we expect the media to live up to its code of ethics.

The press tells, manipulates, suggests, persuades, and orders through messages. Napoleon said, "A hostile newspaper is much more to be feared than a thousand bayonets." Today, the media has a lot of political influence and can, through spoken, printed, or visual expression, change the meaning of an event or modify the use of a word to satisfy its own motives. Words are powerful weapons, convincing us what to do or not to do. Politicians know that by controlling the media they can control the people.

Who owns the media? Usually governments or big capital interests. In this manner, the delivery of news is highly controlled. Censorship may further tighten that control. To maintain a free press, the media requires conscientious surveillance.

Even when governments don't impose censorship, power groups can cause the media to censor itself. For instance, a free-lance journalist writes an in-depth study for a newspaper on the contamination of the local water supply caused by a local industry that advertises in the newspaper. The industry's board of directors retaliates by discontinuing its advertising in the newspaper, which compels the editors to self-censor all similar material in the future. A controversial radio talk show that exposes illegal dealing, political or public officers, or bribes, or that questions religious authorities, will be flooded by complaints and threats, and the station may even be forced to remove the program.

During the military junta in Argentina from 1976 to 1983, over sixty journalists were killed or declared *desaparecidos* (missing persons). A high toll exacted to preserve freedom of the press. In America, freedom of the press is taken for granted. Except for sporadic book banning by local libraries, we have access to an incredible amount of information from all over the world. What a contrast this is with the Soviet Union or other countries that exert tight control over what can or cannot be published.

Whatever we read, see, or hear, we must question how much of it is information, how much misinformation. It is frightening to think that the media lies to us, but I have some remedies for it. One is to switch off the news. Some have already done it. According to UNESCO, in 1985, it is known or believed that no daily general newspapers are published in thirty-two countries and territories. The same source reports twenty countries or territories without television. The message is: We are able to live without news.

The other, perhaps more practical, remedy against misinformation is to educate ourselves as to the trustworthy sources of unbiased news. Read between the lines. Don't take for granted what you hear or see on TV. Distrust! When I read a paper I keep in mind that the editorial is the opinion of the paper's owner, not necessarily that of the editor. Avoid reading only headlines; the small print may provide a different slant to the story. Try to obtain several sources of information, with different vested interests or ideologies, and sort and compare the reporting in each. Finally, pay attention to who the advertisers are. Their interests are too often reflected in the media they sponsor.

I also consider the subliminal visual medium a potentially dangerous and unacceptable means of communication. It is used to promote commercial products on television and in movies at a level below conscious awareness. Although research has shown this to be largely ineffective for advertising, it may be used to change people's ideologies as well—one reason many countries reject the use of satellites by leading countries to broadcast television programs.

Because we are living in an electronic era, the speed and intensity of much of what we read and hear may exceed our ability to process it. To be integral, we need time for processing and questioning the media information we will store in our brain. In this way, we will preserve ourselves as integral beings.

It is important to discuss the use of torture by government because it threatens the essence of the integral being, the foundation of the family, the validity of society, and the veracity and usefulness of the government itself.

If a government turns into a dictatorship, or is unable to regulate strong dissent, it may resort to unlawful means of control: prison and torture. Of two evils, torture is the worst. Those who have been tortured, or have been in contact with torture victims, know. Torture destroys any value that a society might hold proud. For the victim, the physical pain of torture is mixed with an absolute sense of rejection by God, family, and country. The psychological isolation humiliates our human nature, converting us to defenseless and terrified creatures.

Torture is not on the decline; on the contrary, it is spreading. History has taught us nothing—from Antiochus Epiphanes, King of Syria, who killed and tortured Jews in the second century B.C., to the horrors of the Nazi concentration camps, to the cruel practices of the Shah of Iran's secret police, Savak, we continue to walk territories of desolation, torment, and pain. The cruelty of man has remained unchanged. There are people who make a living inventing devices to torture our minds and bodies. There are companies that sell them. There are physicians whose goal is not to heal, but to keep victims alive so they can be tortured to the limits of their endurance.

In 1972, in my psychiatric research ward in Buenos Aires, I treated a male patient suffering from auditory hallucinations and severe paranoid symptoms. He spoke incessantly and nonsensically of a machine in his throat. No one knew who he was or where he came from. After two months of treatment, he finally gave us his name and we were able to locate his mother. She told us that he had been working as an immigrant laborer in a small town in a neighboring country. Since he owned a small television set and a stereo, the local police had framed him as a thief so they could steal his belongings. He was placed in a concentration camp.

After two years of intensive therapy, the man was able to explain how the guards of the concentration camp tortured him. He was hung from the *pan de arara* (parrot's perch). Then, slowly, he was lowered into a cattle drinking dish while shocks were administered to his neck with the *picana electrica* (cattle prod). Only then was I able to understand what he had meant by having a "machine" in his throat.

According to the 1983 report of Amnesty International, an organization awarded the 1977 Nobel Prize of Peace, 123 countries have abused human rights. Two world-leading countries were among those listed, the United States and the Soviet Union. Human rights violations are a political issue because they involve governments; they are an individual issue because they infringe upon the basic right of freedom.

In countries where the governments are strong, it may not be necessary to jail, torture, or kill us in order to keep things under control. Instead, other means of control are implemented. A government, its institutions, or its social agencies can harass us in our jobs, deny us work, refuse our applications to enter college, audit our income taxes. If we are public figures, our names can be slandered. Ultimately, if a government needs to control the whole country, it may trigger a war to divert attention from the real issues that trouble the country.

If we look into history, the world has always been at war. The reasons for this are multiple and complex; there is no single theory of war. Understanding of war might be grasped after understanding the nature of mankind, a task still unfinished. Wars can fulfill political, territorial, economic, cultural, or religious needs. Both limited and generalized wars kill and destroy; the quantity of the damage is the only difference. To mitigate so much war horror, international laws have been passed. Truly a naïve remedy for barbarous acts.

War is an act of aggression. The public message is, "We must defend ourselves," while the hidden message is, "We must make a profit for those who promote wars." In 1986, the world's military expenditures amounted to almost 812 billion dollars. If someone says, "We must defend our land," I always ask, "Whose land?" Most of us can hardly obtain a mortgage, most of us rent from the rich, and many in the world live in shanties or in the streets. A war gives us orphans, kills our youth, demolishes our houses and factories, and brings famine and disease. As individuals, we cannot escape from this truth.

What can we do to put a stop to so much misery?

Until mutual respect becomes the norm among individuals, and eventually the rule among nations, I doubt we can drastically influence the chronic course of war. Nonetheless, the people of any country should have the right to a plebiscite. We should at least have our voice and vote recorded to choose between war and peace.

If a government has absolute power it will control absolutely. Juvenal, in first-century Rome, said it most succinctly: "Who guard the guardians?"

Assuming we all live in a democratic society, we should have political parties of different ideologies. Thus, different voices will have a chance to be heard if their representatives are elected. A pluralistic system tacitly keeps the official party in check and will restrain those officers who are prone to corruption or are grossly inept. The media, by exposing pitfalls, bribing, and serious wrongdoing, is also a good monitor of government function. Finally, we have our vote to approve or disapprove government actions.

A vote is still the best answer to bad government. However, if it, too, fails, we still have other resources: we can strike, or we can call in a leader.

We have the capacity to stop the world. By a general strike. Can you imagine? The whole world becomes paralyzed. Soldiers, professionals, laborers, business persons, farmers, students—every single human on strike. Violence is stopped, mass media is silenced, factories are closed, electricity is cut off. The whole planet is shut down for one day. A day in which we get close to nature and the universe. A day in which we prove how important we are as individuals.

The right to strike should exist because it is the only way we can demand rights denied us. Even if a strike is illegal, an individual still has the right to walk out. We must remember that individuals should always serve themselves first, then the master.

Barring a strike, a new leader can emerge. Leaders bring about important changes in politics, religions, economics, technology, music, literature, and so forth. The world as we know it is the result of the work of a few individuals who have shaped the course of history. Among them, political leaders occupy a prominent place because their actions help build or destroy countries or whole social systems.

An authentic leader comes to us with certainty, programs, promises, and, most of all, charisma. Charisma is a mixture of charm, mystery, and confidence that says, "Trust me, I am your savior." A leader is born of the people and operates with the people until he or she reaches power.

Confucius, Jesus, Moses, Mohammad, Napoleon, Lincoln, Hitler, Gandhi, Perón, Ho Chi Minh, Castro, and Martin Luther King, Jr., were leaders who made their way up, representing good, evil, or both. Leaders tend to address crowds because credibility already exists in crowds, which do not think or question on a deep level. Hitler, Mussolini, and Perón spoke from balconies while the crowd congregated below. Nowadays, the leader addresses the crowd by television and someone else writes the speech. To look good on the screen, the leader wears makeup. Times change, and so do customs, but the essence of leadership does not.

Leaders appear as models of a desirable social ideal: they have power, knowledge, and fame. We are enticed by their charisma, and we welcome their urge to take care of us. When the society is diseased, it becomes more dependent. A leader fulfills our need for dependency, and becomes the healer of the social system. At a psychological level, leaders represent parental figures because they promise to assume full responsibility for the country's sufferings. How wonderful it is to have a parent again! Going back to ancient times, we see that the Roman leaders were intuitively aware of this when they gave the people bread and circuses.

Although leaders are unavoidable, integral beings must be aware that it is wrong to allow one individual to control the destiny of a country. Integral beings want as little governmental interference as possible in their lives. The brilliance of the individual is systematically dimmed by those who rule to control. Integral beings are left with the dilemma that exists between the individual and the state—both need to be free to control.

Juan Perón emerged as the result of years of oligarchical rule and the undistributed wealth of post–World War II Argentina. After being voted in in democratic elections, he industrialized the country. Although he did not touch the wealth of the rich, he gave to the poor. In fact, he taught the poor about their social rights and brought a sense of national pride to Argentina. Nevertheless, he became dogmatic and dictatorial as a social reformer, and a fascistic form of government developed. In order to obtain a public job one had to be a member of Perón's Justicialista party. Censorship was imposed, intellectuals were persecuted, and dissidents jailed.

What Perón gave to the people he eventually took away. Although he was first a military man, he had the charisma of an extraordinary politician. But more than a politician he was a great psychologist of the people. After his overthrow, he gathered the rich, the middle class, and the poor, the extreme right and left wings, the pious, and the atheistic to make a comeback, eighteen years later.

We are living in a world that tells us to be honest, to work hard, pay our taxes, and love peace. Meanwhile, some rulers and the news media worship and promote rampage, justify violence, and condone immorality. What are we to do? Sit back and enjoy what is available? Look the other way? Keep denying our oppressive reality, hoping our children will have it better?

Not me. I want better things now. I did not come to this earth only to pave the way for other generations. I want my share of this planet. I mean to obtain the right to be healthy, self-sufficient, and capable of using the good things of this earth.

Three factors become obstacles on the road to true democracy: fear, social selfishness, and indifference. A diseased government contaminates societies and families alike. We cannot avoid becoming fearful. As long as our fear remains intact, we will remain slaves unable to accept the challenge of our lives.

Someone once said to me, "I don't care about the state of the world, it doesn't affect me a bit." This is social selfishness, reflecting a serious inability to face the tragic reality of our society. We are not living in isolation; we live within a community of men, women, and children.

Indifference is dangerous because it maintains the status quo. We may remain free by moving toward a democracy of individuals aware of what real freedom for all means. We should demand, as individuals participating in the system, the delivery of freedom, justice, and equality.

Do I go out, then, and fight for my rights? Yes, I will go out, but to become an integral being. In the small triangle of myself, I will develop the qualities I would like to see present in the large triangle of my family, society, and government. As integral beings we must be actively involved in public affairs. We cannot expect others to look after us. Once our diapers are no longer necessary, our responsibilities begin. No matter who is in power, we are responsible for ourselves.

Chapter Five

THE SMALL TRIANGLE

> Then at last there was a man; and Prometheus, son of Iapetos, is said to have taken earth, mixed it with running water, and formed it in the image of the gods that rule the universe.
>
> Ovid, *Metamorphoses*, I, 80

It has been estimated that seventy-five billion people have died in the last million years—and we know that each one of them was a triangle composed of body, intellect, and emotions, as we are.

We are also movement that carries energy and mass, the same energy and mass we find in a handful of soil or a bucket of water. We all are made of atoms, as are sea water and the earth's crust, the same atoms that may one day destroy us. Hence, the biblical observation that we are made of clay is still true.

For the last six hundred million years, the evolution of living organisms has continued. Over 250,000 flower species, thousands of animals, a million or more different species of insects, and ourselves have evolved through natural selection.

It has taken mankind ten to twelve million years to evolve to modern times. One to two and a half million years ago, we became *Homus erectus*. The transition from walking on all fours to two feet was most important. Standing erect, we freed our hands: we started to make objects and to build. We conquered the natural limits of geography by being able to walk, to run, to ride, to climb. The coming of *Homo sapiens*, 350,000 years ago, introduced the quest for knowledge and moral values. Then we had the foundation of a human being: muscle, knowledge, and morals.

Biological evolution takes place through genes and is inherited, while psychosocial evolution is not. It took millions of years of biological evolution to make a human being, and less than fifty years of psychosocial evolution to produce nuclear weapons, invent television, transplant organs, and travel to other planets. Psychosocial evolution happens so rapidly it does not give us a chance to adjust. We become overwhelmed.

Technology may go against the natural laws of this planet by causing a loss of balance. We antagonize nature by creating an artificial milieu in which to live. Today we may choose to live in any land with great variations of temperatures but be warm or cool, and we can eat not only nuts and fruits but artificially created foods. To improve our living conditions, we have perfected technology and put the ecological balance of the earth in jeopardy. The pollution in the air and water, and our diets are poisoning our bodies. Sperm banks are reporting a 30 percent decrease in the male sperm count, which may indicate a trend toward sterility. This decrease has been steadily observed during the last twenty years, which connects it to environmental pollution and radiation.

In a very short period of time we have technologically covered centuries. Is this progress for the better? I believe it is the quality rather then the quantity of life that counts. Our life span has been lengthened, but what good is it to live in fear for seventy years?

I often go to the railroad station and take a seat on one of the wooden benches and watch the anonymous people moving in and out of trains. Where are they coming from? What is their destination? The pace is fast; there is a hypnotic quality that lures me to mix with the crowd. I know for sure that all of us are spinning together with the earth. How can each of us find our individuality?

At the age of ten, before the era of television, I used to accompany one of my uncles, a politician, on his electoral campaign. From a wooden platform raised on street corners or in squares, he would address the crowd. He was tall to my eyes, and taller on the platform. I also remember the parish priest speaking from the pulpit. Before him I felt even smaller. Once I listened to Perón, speaking from the balcony of Casa Rosada, or the "Pink House," as hundreds of thousands cheered him.

It seems to me that most of us are satisfied to mingle in a railroad station. Few of us will stand up on political platforms or in pulpits. And even fewer will become individuals and emerge from the crowd.

One way to remain independent, though, is to keep reminding ourselves that no one owns justice, freedom, and morals exclusively. As long as we don't invade someone else's privacy we have the right to practice our beliefs.

It is a law of nature that for a normal development, a normal environment is required. If we create an abnormal environment—for example, nuclear disaster—we will become abnormal. In this order of things, biological evolution has modified and improved our thinking process, but not our morality. We have been clubbing other human beings for entire epochs, with no relief in sight. Do we have to wait another million years to change? Was Tagore right when he said, "Man is good, but men are not?"

In the brain, we know where the center of rage is and of a chemistry that triggers or inhibits it. Yet no one knows of a center that controls our morals, nor do we know of the existence of a chemistry that checks the moral code. Are we motivated to improve our morals? Do we need to be motivated? And by whom?

Why are we not taught that each of us is unique?

Why has no one ever said to me that my freedom belongs to me? I don't want to be a robot, born to please parents, teachers, and the system. I want to know the truth so I can be free and helpful and loving.

Why doesn't the school curriculum include the teaching of becoming a true individual? Why is the history I was taught not the history that was?

Why do we kill on behalf of God, if we have not yet rationally proved the existence of God? Do we believe in God? Do we live by God's rules?

Do we really believe in anything?

How is it that, with such a God-fearing population, we have so much aggression and corruption?

Are we forced to believe in order to conform with others, to obtain personal gains, or as part of our customary package of survival? What is the difference between Christian morality and other morality? What is Western civilization? What is the first, the second, the third, the fourth, the fifth world?

Questions and no answers. We need to learn. And that means we must reject an educational system that teaches us how to serve the world rather than how to become ourselves.

Are we only a biochemical entity? Are we only a highly organized, complex cellular structure? We are a hundred billion cells, and each cell contains millions of atoms. We come from clay, a kind of clay able to create a symphony or a poem!

We are the sum of the sides of the triangle of body, intellect, and emotions. If one side of the triangle is ill, the other two will be affected because all three sides act in synchrony, adjusting to the side that is off balance. Therefore, all three sides will become ill in order to remain in balance, even if this means "an ill balance."

For example, one has a leg pain caused by the sciatic nerve. By limping, the position of the hip and the leg is changed, and gait becomes abnormal. Now it becomes a medical problem: the sciatic pain and the limping. A doctor decides on hospitalization; X rays show a serious disk problem. Now we are in traction, still in pain, and unable to walk or work. Now we have a social problem. The pain shortens our attention span; immobilization makes us irritable, emotionally unstable. We have to treat the pain with painkillers, perhaps have corrective surgery for our disk problem, have an insurance policy to cover our temporary disability, and have psychological support to accept the setback. Nature, government, society, family, and individual are inextricably interconnected.

I want to be an integral being. Therefore, I must develop my brain to full capacity, bringing out its yet unidentified functions. I must keep myself in shape by having a flexible, well-tuned body. I must control my behavior and shield myself from stress. I must live by my principles, respecting my fellow creatures and nature as I respect myself. Only then will I be an integral being, in balance with family and society.

Is the aim of becoming integral a grandiose proposal? I don't think so. I am not proposing to discover the secret of eternal life. I am only asking to be free, to be healthy, and to live with dignity. Yet these intentions are hard ones to fulfill. It requires a lot of work, discipline, and sacrifice. I have no time to waste. I have to do it here and now.

Within the context of the universe, we are a small miracle, which we overlook with our arrogance. To become an integral being we need humility to accept and take care of the miracle we are. Our aim is to become a single unity within the world. Inner and Outer knowledge, health, and freedom will become available. We will develop techniques to acquire new habits, to wake up dormant emotions, to reshape body parts, to nurture body and intellect.

Here is a list of attributes required to become an integral being: acceptance, acculturation, adjustability, courage, education, emotionality, endurance, health, honesty, know-how, love, mutual respect, sacrifice, self-awareness, self-discipline, self-limitation, tolerance, and trust.

Whether we are a colony of cells or the creation of a supreme being, we are what we see: a sum of systems. From the union of an ovule and a spermatozoon, we develop a body entrusted to us by nature so we can complete our mission on earth. Our body is sacred, like all those things we love and care for. At the outset of life, we are confined to our cribs and to the arms of our parents. It takes about ten months before we are able to crawl, twelve to take our first step. At this point, the universe begins to open up for us. When we begin to walk away from the crib, the long walk toward loneliness starts. We have a need to be free, yet we learn very fast the meaning of the word *no*. We are caught between our dependency on our parents and our need for others. We start to socialize, learn how to share, and explore our own sexuality.

As adolescents our idols are no longer our parents but someone else—a movie star, a sports hero, a famous singer. We identify with beauty, strength, and wealth. It is a volcanic age—the breast in the girl, the beard in the boy, the first menstruation, the first ejaculation.

Adolescence is a time of doubt, of dreams, of hopes. The social pressure is great; the peer group demands uniformity of behavior—the same hairdo, the same slacks, the urge to have it all, now. And so what began as a true individual, the body who was master of the world, now becomes the slave of social rules.

Between the ages of twenty and twenty-two, our bodies stop growing. The woman has soft lines, her breast is a symbol of food, of eroticism, an aesthetic component of her life. The man has muscles and a beard. At this age, we complete the development of our character, the way we act and react. Our behavior and habits are well established, and we show a specific profile of our mind: the persona.

We begin to time life's course according to the watch. We have particular habits of grooming, arranging objects, a taste for certain foods, hobbies, and other interests. All these components make us who we are. In addition, the silent language of our body gestures, posture, walk adopts its own individuality and becomes part of us.

By now we know what we really want to be. We choose a trade, a profession; we must be self-sufficient. We are ready to form a family, if that is our desire. At this time in our life, excuses are no longer valid; we ought to have goals, respect life, demand our rights, abide by our duties. Therefore, we must develop a system of self-defense to preserve our body and identity. We must develop a strategy to enable us to attain what we want: to fulfill our needs and be happy. It is tough out there. Family and society are very demanding and practical when it comes to their needs. All our dreams and ideals will fall short of the target when confronted with forces looking after their own interests.

The integral being must have appeared by this stage. Lawful, strong, understanding but defiant, we don't allow anyone to step on us. If we do not become integral beings, we will walk into middle age as the term indicates, in the middle—half strong, half healthy; half happy, half defeated.

At forty-five we should have a pretty good idea of what has happened to us. The decline of our kingdom has become quite evident: we lose our hair or our waistlines; we need more light to read; we get closer to the mirror to shave. Our skin and hopes begin to sag. So we decide to take a break in our long life journey and look back.

What do we see? Success and failure, sorrow and happiness, remorse and hatred, anger and peace. We may then decide to conform; now it is a matter of survival. A tremendous fear of losing what we have and of being unable to obtain anything further from life pervades.

Do not give up. I have no difficulty accepting the fact that I am a middle-aged man. I feel no uneasiness telling anyone that life has been hard, and that I have lost when I thought I was a winner, that I went through a divorce when the marriage was "perfect," that it was incredibly painful to tell five children that Daddy was leaving home. But I never gave up, even when I lost my position at the hospital. I kept on fighting, discussing, organizing. It was the toughest time of my life. Fifteen years later, I am back on my feet and remarried. But I still make a point to respect the beliefs and behaviors of others. And I am still a rebel.

Middle age is a myth, like all other ages. Inside, we never age. It is society that ages us prematurely. We age at forty-five simply because we are expected to age then. If we are in good integral health we will age later in life—if at all. Nature has trusted us with our body. Have we honored that trust?

How do we define an old person? Is an old person one who has given up the zest for life? As long as we have a future ahead of us, dreams to think of, and motivations to keep us interested, we are not old.

I am happy to say that I have a future. Because I still have places to go, dreams and projects to fulfill. I envision many years ahead during which I expect to reach new goals. I am getting older, but I still like to be pampered, taken care of, being a child once in a while. I don't mind it when my aunt Elena knits a sweater for me. When I go back to Buenos Aires, I eat familiar dishes, gaze at old pictures, ask questions about my childhood, my mother.

Old people are wonderful. They carry a tremendous amount of love, knowledge, and an unbeatable dignity. I hope that I will always have someone older than myself in my life.

If I allow myself to be pessimistic, skeptical, envious, or cynical, only looking at the negative side of life, I will age rapidly. Many my age talk about nothing but their children's achievements, instead of their own. There is no future ahead of them. They live vicariously through their children.

Becoming old is also a serious matter. It is then that we begin to complete our earthly destiny—from dust to dust. We have slowed down in our long walk. Due to dehydration, our height has lost an inch or so. Our senses have lost their keen edge. We are more frugal; we need less sleep. Yet, because we don't seek out competition or rivalry we are more accepting of others. Although our memory starts to vanish, the memory of childhood and younger years comes back with intensity and nostalgia. Sometimes we invent a more benign past, and that is fine. The final years are arriving; it is now when we look into our origins.

Why are we here? Are we on earth to explain our ignorance? Are we on earth, as anything else is in the universe, to preserve its continuity? It is easier to explain an atom and its presence on earth than to offer a reasonable explanation for our own existence. We are here for a purpose. Could it be to destroy nature, as we are currently doing? It is more sensible to see our presence on this planet as part of a larger pattern, searching for completeness. Is Earth a way station among many other interplanetary stations? Are we here as part of a reincarnation?

I'd rather be an active voyager on our cosmic trip than be a bystander. We are already submerged in the gusts of space, time, and energy. We are already whirling, circling, flooding the territory of our lives. We cannot escape; we are here to stay.

We can actively participate in the continuous process of nature's interactions if we integrate. Isolation drives us into a chronic and negative loneliness. We should have insight into our imcompleteness and our human limitations, so we can grow and develop.

Krishnamurti, the Indian philosopher, said that when the mind is completely aware we become silent. In our awareness, thoughts do not intervene; we are observers of our own thoughts, of our own movements and actions. We move out of our small triangle and watch ourselves. Then we are ready for change. When things go wrong, we always have the option to change or not. In spite of serious setbacks, people can adapt to change.

Most of us would like the world to change instead of us. One of my tasks as a psychiatrist is to offer my patients programs that will alter their lives. Most patients want changes overnight. One was twenty-three years old, a college dropout, religious, working part-time in a grocery store. One night she overdosed on tranquilizers. Her depression had started at eighteen. In a period of five years she had consulted four psychiatrists, two psychologists, had had one hospital admission for attempted suicide, one abortion, heavy marijuana use, and a father killed in a car accident. Now she wanted to "really" change.

After I examined her I explained that she should make a second appointment, so we could discuss her test findings and write a treatment program. She said that she wanted treatment right then and there. "Why do I have to come back?" she said to me, perplexed. I told her that what she needed was a complete overhaul, which could not be performed instantly.

I never saw her again. Her attitude was typical of many patients and people in general. They want magic to obtain instant relief.

In *A Course in Miracles,* published by the Foundation for Inner Peace, I read, "Nothing real can be threatened, nothing unreal exist." Yet we feel threatened. We create around us a world of unreality that is indeed threatening. Consequently, we are prone to distrust. The remedy for unreasonable distrust is love. In love we find safety and peace, an acceptable definition of God. Thus, if we are loving and peaceful we can be gods ourselves. We are all part of the universe, and what is God but an expanding universe? Each of us is on this earth to become an integral being, to acquire a sense of belonging, of universal oneness. Perhaps we are gods, linked to the vastness of the universe.

When we are old, we are ready to leave this earth. Integral old people have a special kind of dignity and pride, summarizing an exemplary life. Their mission is accomplished. We find this in their eyes, perhaps because, as the ancients used to say, the eyes are the mirrors of the soul.

··· *Chapter Six*

THE BODY

> I love your body.
>
> > Overheard in the
> > New York City subway

The first time I was in a funeral parlor the corpse appeared in better health than the mourners. Our need to disguise death and prolong our stay on this earth, even after death, has been candidly expressed throughout history. Body preservation was customary in ancient cultures like those of the Egyptians and the Incas and Paracas of Peru. We have built cities for the dead and devised lavish burial ceremonies. In the Pacific, burial practices take up to one year. We can be buried in the ground, in the ocean, or be put out to dry in the open. Some cultures have eaten their enemies to gain strength; others have eaten their relatives to sooth grief. So many ways of handling the dead, and often so costly! Wouldn't it be better to pay as much attention to our living bodies?

    The Greeks worshipped strong, beautiful bodies. Their sculpture remains as a living testimony. For the warrior, the body was a symbol of strength, for the slaver, an object for sale. Yet the more humanity became interested in religion, the more the body became related to sin. Redemption consisted of punishing bodies with whips and fasting. Fashion also led to punishment. At the beginning of this century, romantic attitudes favored pale, thin, weak bodies. To obtain this physical state, one had to eat little and become careless in matters of health. It was considered chic for a woman to faint. Tuberculosis, which was represented as loss of weight and coughing up blood, was viewed to some degree as a "romantic illness."

Although the first human autopsy was performed by Herophilus in Alexandria in 300 B.C., autopsies in the Middle Ages were banned on religious grounds and misconceptions about the human body flourished. It was believed that the bone of resurrection was located in the big toe, that the Adam's rib really was missing, and that the heart had a long-lasting bone.

More than two hundred anatomical errors were made by Galen and carried over the centuries by his disciples. But they were corrected by one man, Andreas Vesalius of Belgium. In 1537, at the age of twenty-three, Vesalius began to unveil the secrets of the human body, and, thereafter, great progress was made in understanding anatomy and its functions.

Technical advancements, however, have not been reflected in our personal interest in our bodies. To let anatomists, physiologists, or physicians do the job is all right, but not enough. We think of the body as a car. We believe we don't need to know a lot about it, nor do we wish to, as long as we can drive it. We buy the gas, the oil, and we go to the mechanic for repairs. But when a car gets old, we sell it or dump it. We cannot do that with our body— we are stuck with it for life.

To become integral beings, it is essential to have solid knowledge of our bodies. Any attempts to disassociate ourselves from our bodies should be immediately rejected. Learning about anatomy and the way body parts function will help us keep them fit.

I am startled by the human body because it is not only beautiful but intriguing. Although all human bodies are alike, faces and voices are not. There are billions of us, yet we are all different. Whether I am the temple of God, my own temple, the greatest lover on earth, or a hospital record, I am myself—unique. I know I have a body that I must tolerate and vice versa. I wish to get to know my body, I wish to prevent disease and avoid a premature death. Without my body, I don't count in my connection to the universe and nature.

I watch people. Their posture, gait, weight, wrinkles, gestures give cues. As a physician, examining the human body unfolds information related to heritage, predisposition to illness, personality traits, and even socioeconomic background. The body is a walking autobiography.

There is nothing wrong about undressing to look at oneself, to feel our skin, muscles, and bones, or to buy a stethoscope to listen to the sound of our heart. Looking in a mirror, we may say, "Is that all there is?" That is because we are seeing our body *image*, which may not be related to the way our body really is. Close your eyes for a moment and try to visualize your body. Think of your posture—whether you are standing, sitting, or crossing your legs. Obese or anorectic people may not perceive their bodies as others perceive them. Handsome or ugly people have different perceptions of their own handsomeness or ugliness. It is essential that we each accept our body as it is, in its shape, texture, and smell.

• • •

The Insiders

In the Koran, it says, "Does man think we shall never put his bones together again? Indeed, we can remold his very fingers."

Did you realize that without bones we would collapse? Thank goodness we have 209 indistinct bones. The skeleton holds us together, takes us places, works with us, and protects our organs from injury. The brain, which is so fragile, is safely encased in the skull. Bones are live tissue; in their marrow the white cells of the blood, which help fight disease, are born. The enamel of the teeth is the hardest of all human tissue and lasts longest after death.

Many human diseases affect the bones, leaving imprints that last forever. These imprints allow archeologists to determine how long an illness has existed around the world. Even psychological stress may leave its trademark in our bones.

When the news reports that the government is employing a "muscle-flexing policy," we know what it means: force. We have always fantasized about force: Atlas holding the world on his shoulders, Samson demolishing a temple, or modern man lifting 1,411 pounds. Yet muscles are more than force; they are movement—clearly shown in record-breaking performances like swimming at 4.39 miles per hour or running at 26.5 miles per hour. Muscles are 43 percent of our body weight. Wherever there is movement, there is muscle, even in the lungs, stomach, or arteries. Although we think of muscles as mechanical components, they also participate in our emotional life every time we tense up or smile.

Ligaments, tendons, cartilage, and skin provide support for our organs. Spreading throughout the body, fat helps contour them and protect them from changes in outside temperatures. Fatty tissue is present around and inside the heart and liver. Keep in mind that in obesity, fat increases in every organ.

Few words in the human vocabulary have the emotional force of *heart* and *blood*. Human heart sacrifices, the heartaches of lovers, bloodthirsty gods and vampires, the warrior offering his blood are vivid images and associations.

The heart is a pump that weighs, in adults, between 8 and 12 ounces. It carries blood to the lungs and to the rest of the body. It beats about 72 times per minute, but it may go faster or slower, according to the body's needs for blood and oxygen. The pace is also related to the size of the pump. In elephants, the heart beats about 25 times per minute, while in birds it beats 1,000 times per minute. In general, in twenty-four hours the heart pumps the equivalent of 2,642 gallons of blood to a network of arteries, veins, and capillaries that constitute a distance of 60,000 miles. The width of the arteries varies from one hundredth of an inch in the smallest capillary to one inch in the aorta.

There are a group of arteries that are very dear to us—the coronaries. Emotional and reflecting extremes, I call them the arteries of our soul. Excessive stress, smoking, drinking, poor dietary habits, and lack of physical exercise will eventually clog our coronaries and result in a heart attack.

On October 30, 1983, at 6 P.M., I had a heart attack. Although I only had symptoms of indigestion I knew I was having it. (I suppose it was my medical intuition.) I asked my wife to drive me to Winthrop University Hospital in Mineola, New York. As she wheeled me into the emergency room, I noticed that after forty-nine years I was in a stroller again. Then, nurses took off my trousers and I felt defenseless, my Latin macho symbol stripped away. A priest asked me whether I wanted the last rites. (Was I going to engage myself, as was customary, in a theological argument?)

My physician confirmed my diagnosis. He would try to dissolve the clot lodged in one of the coronary arteries by injecting an enzyme. I signed the authorization for the procedure.

I remember being completely without fear, yet extremely concerned about my wife and five children. When the operation began, I saw my deceased mother and an unknown lady sitting at the foot of my bed. There was no wall beyond them and my bed, only open space. Was I dreaming? No. I had had a cardiac arrest. I was clinically dead. I opened my eyes and knew I didn't want to come back. I thought I had found absolute peace.

But it was then I decided not to give up. So strong was the image of my wife and children that I fought back, along with the help of the wonderful staff that took care of me. The procedure was successful, the clot was dissolved. Further testing showed no heart damage.

The next morning I came to realize the duality of life and death. How quick the transition between them is!

In Aristotle's time, it was believed that blood moved in an ebb and flow, like the sea. In the sixteenth century, the English anatomist William Harvey discovered that blood circulates. Each of us has about five liters of it that circulates to feed the tissues, remove waste, carry heat, and defend us from infection. The blood has red cells to carry oxygen, white cells to destroy bacteria and poisons, and platelets to repair vessel walls and form clots to prevent leaking. Sugar, vitamins, fats, proteins, minerals, and hormones circulate in the blood wherever they are needed.

Our cardiovascular system responds promptly to any sign of alarm. In case of mental or physical threat our arteries contract, our heart beats faster, and blood is rapidly sent wherever it is required. Our cardiovascular system assists us in our physical, emotional, and intellectual journey, carrying life to each one of our cells.

Our lungs are two bellows located in the chest. They are pink at birth but may, due to pollution or smoking, be black during adulthood. The function of the lungs is to exchange oxygen and carbon dioxide with the air we breathe. This air arrives at the lungs after traveling through our nasal cavity, throat, larynx, trachea, and bronchi.

One would think that because breathing is essential to our lives, a lot of interest would be paid to the way we do it. Yet we had to wait until 1777 when Antoine-Laurent Lavoisier, a French chemist, became interested in respiration. In the lungs, there are 300 to 400 million alveoli, which are the units of respiration. These alveoli are in direct contact with the capillaries, exchanging gases from and to the blood. Breathing is automatically controlled by changes occurring in brain centers. We breathe about fourteen times per minute, using fourteen pints of air per minute. The deeper we breathe, the better off we are. Unfortunately, most of us breathe too shallowly. The ribs and muscles of the chest are needed to expand and contract the lungs. A well-developed chest will help us breathe better.

Breathing is also related to our emotions. Some people hold their breath for a few moments to relieve their anxiety; others breath very fast. If we deprive brain cells of oxygen for eight minutes, the cells die and the damage is irreversible. The record for a man going without oxygen is five minutes.

The digestive system processes, absorbs, and uses food, and finally rids the body of its waste. At first food is cut, torn, crushed, and ground by our teeth. It is then mixed, by our tongue, with saliva, which contains enzymes. These enzymes, which are also found along the digestive tract, are chemicals that break the food down into small particles for absorption in the stomach, where the food gets mixed with gastric juice.

The heavier the meal, the longer the food stays in the stomach; for example, a five-hour stopover is required for pork. After that, it's ready to go through the twenty feet of small intestine, where absorption begins to take place through 350 square yards of villi. Through villi we absorb nutrients and water. In the small intestine, the bile of the liver and other enzymes break the food down further. The large intestine, or colon, measures about five feet in length and stores our solid waste. In the colon, colonies of bacteria eat the debris of our food and synthesize some of the vitamins as well. It takes about twenty-four hours for a meal to travel from mouth to rectum. We defecate about ten ounces of feces per day.

The liver is a chemical plant that processes, purifies, and stores substances. The liver is made up of 50,000 to 100,000 filters, or lobules, that purify our blood. It stores vitamins A, B, B-12, D, E, K, sugar, and minerals, including iron and copper. Vitamins A and B-12 can be stored for very long periods of time. This is why an excessive amount of vitamin A may damage the liver. The liver also produces half a liter of blood and half a liter of bile. Bile is needed for the absorption of fats. Below the liver is the gall bladder, a reservoir for the bile.

The pancreas, located behind the stomach, is a gland that secretes digestive enzymes, insulin, and glucagon to regulate the sugars of the body.

The two kidneys are located in the back of the abdomen, in the lower back. The kidneys maintain water and mineral equilibrium. In addition, they filter the impurities of 190 liters of blood per day. The waste products of this metabolism are 1.5 liters of water, which is stored as urine in the bladder. The urine reaches the bladder by two tubes called urethers. We usually urinate about six times per day.

Whatever is not recycled in our bodies is excreted as solid waste, the feces, or as liquid waste, urine and sweat, or in breathing, as gas waste.

In man, the testes are lodged in the scrotum, a pouch of skin lying below the pubis, where they manufacture spermatozoon and male hormones called androgens. The testes are located outside the abdomen because the body heat would kill the spermatozoon. Hence, the scrotum contracts when exposed to cold and expands when exposed to heat.

The spermatozoon are stored as sperm in the seminal vesicle and then conveyed into a main duct, the epididymis, which if untangled, would measure twenty feet. Spermatozoon can be forced out of the body by direct stimulation of the nervous system, or by masturbation or sexual intercourse.

The prostate is very small and lies in front of the rectum. The two ejaculatory ducts enter the prostate and join the urethra, which is the duct that brings to the penis either urine or sperm. On each side of the prostate there is a pear-sized gland that during sexual excitement secretes a liquid that lubricates the prostate.

The ovaries, the sexual glands of the woman, are located in the lower part of the abdomen, one on each side. They produce ova for reproduction and the female hormones estrogen and progesterone. The ovaries are connected to tubes that open in the uterus. The uterus is a muscle with a glandular lining. Once a month, if fertilization of the ova by a spermatozoon does not take place, the lining of the uterus sheds and bleeds. This monthly cycle is called menstruation, and, for unknown reasons, has the same rhythm—twenty-eight days—as the moon's cycle.

The vagina is an elastic canal that communicates to the outside through the vulva, or vaginal entrance. The vulva is surrounded by skin folded into two sets of thick lips called the *labia majora* and *minora*. Beneath the vulva's forward ends, half concealed, is the clitoris. This is an erectile tissue, the equivalent of the male penis. Behind the clitoris is the opening of the urethra. The vaginal entrance is guarded by the hymen, a membrane whose integrity symbolizes virginity. The hymen may be torn during sexual intercourse, intensive physical exercise, or an internal examination.

The nervous system is divided in two parts, central and peripheral. The central nervous system is made up of the brain, cerebellum, pons, medulla oblongata, and the spinal cord. The function of the nervous system is to receive, process, and store information, and to return impulses triggering behavior. The central nervous system is composed of 100 billion cells called neurons. Neurons are made up of "body" and fibers called dendrites and axons. A bundle of axons form nerves, roughly resembling a coaxial cable. Each neuron measures from a fraction of an inch, like those of the brain, to several feet long in the peripheral nerves of tall people. Neurons have difficulty in regenerating after an injury, particularly in the case of brain and spinal cord injuries.

The peripheral nervous system shares some activities with the central nervous system. It innervates the body wall structure and the internal organs, carrying information from the periphery to the brain and vice versa.

In the past thirty years we have heard a lot about the brain because progress has been made in the understanding of how it works, how it becomes ill, and what we can do about it. However, the brain, a soft gray organ with an average weight of 49 ounces, remains intriguing. People used to believe that the bigger the brain, the brighter the person. A blue whale's brain weighs 227 ounces, and the field mouse's brain only 0.018 ounces. Yet, when comparing total body weight to brain weight, man comes first, followed by the dolphin and the field mouse. The adult human brain constitutes only 2 percent of the body weight, while at birth it is 12.4 percent of the body weight. The brain grows rapidly until the age of three, then slows down until the age of seven. Thereafter it continues to grow slowly until the age of twenty, when its final weight is attained.

Although brain cells do not contract, move, divide, or grow further, the brain works. All body functions are regulated by centers located in different regions of the brain. There are motor, sensorial, emotional, and intellectual brain centers. The last is divided into a left hemisphere and a right hemisphere. The left hemisphere of the brain is said to be the seat of logical thought, including inference and language, while performance, mechanical tasks, visual-spatial relationships, creativity, and appreciation of form and color seem to be properties of the right hemisphere of the brain. The right brain controls the motor activity of the left part of our body while the left brain controls the right side. With a brain injury on one side of the brain, we do not become completely paralyzed because the other half of the body remains unaffected.

The brain is fed with oxygen, proteins, carbohydrates, fats, minerals, and vitamins like the rest of our body. Yet the brain needs other foods that will never arrive through the bloodstream: food for the spirit and intellect. These foods may be the sound of music, the reading of poetry, a country view, a change of seasons, an oil painting, a handshake, the loss of a loved one, and, in general, all things that make an emotional, intellectual, or sensorial impact on us. These foods enter our brain, via the senses, to modify the brain's chemical and electrical activity.

The brain is an integrative organ. It has the capacity to absorb an event and chemically store it converted into a memory that years later may be retrieved as a tear. This capacity of the brain to blend, to assimilate chemistry and electricity, pictures and sounds, passions and fears, is amazing enough. But the brain is more than that; it keeps things in harmony. It is a system of tightly intertwined and integrated cells making continuous connections with the rest of our body and the outside world. The brain is a perfect integrative model from which we can learn to become integral beings.

The stillness of a summer night is suddenly interrupted by the chirping of a small cricket. This sound is a lover's mating call. Don't we lower and soften our voices during courtship? What we are doing—us and the crickets—is using the sense of hearing to obtain pleasure through another sensorial experience: sex. The senses give us the basic elements that keep us alert and alive: pleasure and pain.

The senses are organs that receive external and internal inputs and carry them to the brain. Tradition lists five senses: sight, hearing, smell, taste, and touch. We are able to sense temperature, color, light, pain, odors, sounds, and so forth. Sometimes we utilize more than one sense to receive a stimulus—for instance, smell in tasting food. Other times we employ more than one sense to enhance the pleasure of perceiving—the arrangement of a dining table, the color combination of the dishes, and so on. Some people have claimed to see colors when they hear music, or to hear sounds when they see words or images. This phenomenon is called synesthesia, and it is due to the overlapping of impulse transmission. Senses have cell receptors and nerves to send the impulse of stimulus to the brain centers. In the brain, the stimulus is interpreted and processed. Only then does it become a sensation that can be stored in our memory for future reference.

Not everyone perceives a stimulus in exactly the same manner. In burning the tip of a finger with a match, two people will report different degrees of pain. The same happens with the taste of food, musical choices, museum exhibits, or fabric textures. These differences also help us understand our biological individuality, which will help us become integral beings.

Receptors for touch, temperature, and pain are located throughout the skin, distributed in different quantities with varying qualities. We have receptors for soft and hard pressure, warmth and cold. Pain receptors are also located in our inner organs. Pain is a feared experience, the intensity of which varies from person to person. This can be due to our emotional state at the particular time of pain. In the midst of battle, a wounded soldier may not feel pain but will only become aware of it when his senses move from attending to the battle to attending to the wound.

Food presentation, color, smell, taste, and texture tempt us to eat, even when we are not hungry. This reaction is a cooperative function of our senses of sight, taste, smell, and touch. It also shows how our sense organs develop into sophisticated critics of our surroundings if we train them. We use about one million taste buds located in our tongue to distinguish various flavor combinations. From the basic tastes—sweet, bitter, sour, and salty—a wine taster may be able to discriminate more than four hundred variations.

We also use the word *taste* to indicate our ability to dress elegantly, decorate a house, make a flower arrangement, or set a table. Over the centuries, we have developed our senses to interact with our psychological centers. This intricate combination has created the sensuous individual. We see a picture, but we also experience it. It may evoke memories of past experiences, satisfy our aesthetic and emotional needs, stimulate our intellectual cells, or all of these. We want to look pretty, smell good, have soft, velvety skin, taste vintage wines, and dine on superb meals. All these physical and psychological interactions can be repeated every time we dress, eat, make love, go to a museum, attend a concert, or stroll in a park.

Our sensuality is carefully monitored by industries that appeal to our senses to sell products. Advertising is geared to stimulate or change a need. Then it sells the product that will suppress an odor, wash an impurity, scent a room, rejuvenate the skin, offer a glorious dining experience, or even sell a silk-lined casket for a funeral. Billions of dollars are spent to satisfy our senses.

Whether it is a fruity, flowery, spicy, burned, or stale

odor, we smell all the combinations with our olfactory nerve. Scientists have stated that we can differentiate five thousand odors. We all produce normal odors that give us a unique profile. The smell of our body may change during disease or an intense emotional state, such as fear or sexual excitement. As long as we remain clean, our smell is not offensive. Social pressure and commercial interests, however, have fostered a feeling of dirtiness associated with our natural body smell. The perfume industry now promotes musk, an essence reminiscent of our natural sexual scent. Hence, people can purchase a perfume to cancel out their natural one.

Our senses govern our interaction with life in general. The eye continuously records images and colors registering the existing physical world, forcing us to keep in touch with reality. Do we close our eyes to avoid a disturbing image? The eyeball operates like a photographic camera, protected by the eyelids and lubricated by tear glands. Blinking uniformly distributes the tears and washes out dust. But there is much more to blinking. When we walk down a supermarket aisle, for instance, and a product draws our attention, our blinking rate per minute increases. This blinking might even be recorded by a hidden camera, helping a manufacturer to identify potential buyers of a product. Even our eyelids are linked to the socioeconomic system.

If we look inside the eye, we will be able to see the only nerve of the body that is available for inspection, the optic nerve. The eyes are the windows of the brain and, it's true, of our emotions. "Tell me the truth! Look me in the eye!" The first emotional clues are always given away by our eyes.

Hearing starts at the ear, which receives sounds and then responds to them. The ear is divided into three sections:

external, middle, and inner. The external ear is formed by the auricle and the external canal. The auricle is fixed in man, but is mobile in animals, where it helps to collect sound and pinpoint direction. From the auricle the sound moves into the external ear canal, finally to reach the eardrum. When sound hits the eardrum, the central portion of the eardrum vibrates; then part of the sound is rejected and part is absorbed. The absorbed sound is received in the middle ear by a chain of three tiny bones. From there, the sound enters the inner ear, and sensory cells, known as the hair cells, pick it up and send it to the main hearing center of the brain. Sound can also be received through the bone conduction of the skull.

Hearing identifies the sources of sounds and helps us to find direction; it is an important part of our communication system. Strong or loud sounds produce arousal and thus stimulate our bodies. Continuous perception of strong sounds may cause irritability or aggressive behavior. Soft sounds soothe our spirits. Hearing therefore modifies our moods. For the blind, echo sounds, produced by footsteps or the banging of a cane, are used to avoid obstacles.

Whether we hold an epicurean view of pleasure as an ultimate life goal or believe that perception alone is the only valid knowledge, as the Indian Carvakas philosophers of the fourteenth century proposed, we all have senses with which to perceive our world. The senses open the door of our inner self to a world eager to sell us its products. We are attracted to pleasant experiences and often give in to the lures of the environment, but human beings are not ascetics, naturally inclined to refrain from material pleasures. Therefore, we have to caution ourselves from overdoing it. Our senses may lead us up the path to freedom or may entice us into an endless slavery. Although Epictetus of

Hierapolis stated that we may not be responsible for our ideas, we are responsible for the actions resulting from those ideas.

Now that we are at the end of our corporeal journey, we are ready to look in the mirror again. And what do we see? A factory at work, millions of cell workers celebrating life. It is a finished product, the body, although we will cover it with garments. Nonetheless, our face, hands, feet, posture, and walk will give us away. We can hide only so much of our individuality. The wide and flat feet of a peasant, the rigid posture of a soldier, the gaunt face of the terminally ill person, the weathered skin of a farmer, the long, strong hands of a pianist, all denote important aspects of our lives. Throughout our life, our body captures and imprints on itself our physical, emotional, and intellectual makeup. A healthy body is an essential part of becoming an integral being. The most important patrimony is our life. It is up to us to own it and to preserve it in its entirety.

Who are we in these bodies that carry life and death with almost identical defiance? We are those who have perfected destruction to unthinkable details. We are those who have written poems to soothe the sorrow of our race. We are those who dream and fight injustice. We are nature's traveling atoms, visiting all the regions of space, sometimes becoming flesh and bones: our body. Our body, friend and stranger, lover and enemy.

· · · *Chapter Seven*

THE PASSIONS

> And passion, having my best judgement collied.
>
> Shakespeare, *Othello*, III, 3

Within the animal kingdom, we share three primary emotions: fear, rage, and love. These help us, respectively, to flee, fight, and possess. For the social animal, us, there are three more emotions: duty, and, usually hidden, envy and avarice.

All six emotions can reach high levels of intensity and perseverance, hence they are also known as passions. Each of these emotions has its own voice and opinion; they can be very convincing, and, if left uncontrolled, they can dominate our life.

We are on this earth to know, to reason, and to do, but we are also here to feel. As long as we feel, our emotions will impinge on our behavior, causing pleasant or unpleasant responses. Because emotions might overpower reason, integral beings must learn how to identify, feel, express, and master them. Otherwise, uncontrolled emotions may disrupt the making of an integral being.

· · ·

Fear

Do you ever shake when your boss decides to talk to you unexpectedly? Do you know why you cried at birth? Or why you hesitate to say "I love you" even if you know how much you are in love? Do you remember how tall everyone and everything looked when you were a child? Or how you felt when your parents slapped your face? Do you remember when you thought you were going crazy? Do you know why we keep apologizing without knowing the reason? Do you know why when someone died you thought, When will I be dead? Or why some people keep worshipping lies when you ask for the truth, or smile when they should cry, or laugh when they should scream, or are peaceful when they should destroy? Do you remember finding that you know nothing, and in despair, screaming, "Oh, my God!" and then realizing that you fear God as well?

Fear is a response to a threatening stimulus. Through fear, our motor activity and capacity to think become impaired, sometimes to complete immobility, even death. Fear is an alarm system that warns us of an impending danger, although that danger might not be seen as such by others. Someone who is afraid to use an elevator because it may break and fall, for instance.

In my psychiatric practice, fear is a daily visitor. I see three main causes: fear of the unknown, fear of losing one's reason, and fear of losing one's freedom. These three fears mold our lives and shape our fate, but we hardly talk about them, even to ourselves. Why do we silence these fears? Do we do it out of shame? Is it because we accept them as inherited handicaps, or as the reality of our social condition? When we don't know, we suffer the uncertainty, the anxiety, provoked by the unexpected—we fear.

The sources of fear that threaten our everyday life are authority, disease, pain, failure, loneliness, separation, ridicule, rejection, poverty, catastrophe, death, war, and revolution. All these causes threaten our integrity and our happiness. With each, we face the possibility of losing health, love, and/or money.

Fear also affects us physically, because we have a physical site of fear. It is located in the hypothalamus, a region of the brain linked to our emotional life. The hypothalamus is related to sex, sleep, thirst, sugar metabolism, blood pressure, and rage. The autonomic nervous system, which coordinates our body functions, also responds to frightening situations with physical symptoms: cold, clammy hands, excessive perspiration, hand tremors, facial twitches, dry mouth, tightening of the jaws, difficulty in swallowing, butterflies in the stomach, heartburn, diarrhea, nausea, frequent urination, irregular heartbeat, high or low blood pressure, dizziness, and muscle tension.

The physical symptoms of fear can also be experienced without the participation of psychological or external stimuli. If we inject ourselves with epinephrine, a substance normally present in our body, we will experience symptoms resembling fear. It is useful to keep this in mind when we experience fear without apparent reason because it may have a biological cause.

The severity of fear is indicated by duration and intensity. A sudden fear will produce a short, frightened response, but a long-lasting fear will produce a fearful individual. The latter is the more serious consequence, affecting the whole life of the person.

Intensity determines the stages of fear. The first stage is anxiety, usually controllable by medication or relaxation exercises. If mild, most people accept it as it is. If fear cannot be kept under control, we will experience an advanced state of fear known as panic. During a panic attack, we can no longer reason; we behave like automatons. Some undesirable accidents, such as bladder or rectal incontinence or fainting, may result. In severe cases, we may go into convulsions. An example of a panic attack is the case of the war "hero" who runs toward the enemy line and overpowers a machine gun outpost when he is actually panicking. After panicking, we hardly remember anything. The end result of fear is terror. During terror, we become motionless. We are "in shock." If the fear is overwhelming, we can even die.

Producing fear has been the most important action utilized by human forces to control or enslave human beings throughout history. Fear has influenced the destinies of countries and their people. Wars, dictatorships, torture, and the concept of religious hell illustrate the preponderance of fear as a ruling force. Nevertheless, people rarely admit to being frightened. Because fright is shameful and socially unacceptable. By concealing fear, we deny ourselves the opportunity to obtain assistance during our frightening experience or state.

We should make a clear distinction between a frightened person and a fearful person. A frightened person has a transient fear that will come and go. A fearful person lives continuously in fear. A fearful person has an urge to check on causes of fear and is obsessed with the inability to cope with threatening stimuli. That person fears fear itself. In the fearful person fear is glued to the personality in such a way that no one will be able to distinguish that person from fear itself.

There are coping mechanisms to deal with fear. First, we have to learn about it. When did we become acquainted with fear? At the moment we cried for the first time, when our parents first said no, when we got a gentle slap on our hand for reaching out to a hot stove? We learn about fear in school, when we are punished, when we are isolated for physical, social, or economic reasons. We learn about fear, when we must be on our own and have to bargain for our own place on this earth.

Second, we have to establish whether our fear is reasonable or unreasonable.

Third, we have to examine vague fears and analyze them. Many times we question the reasons for our fright and don't get an answer. Some fears are deeply hidden in ourselves, and we would do well to do a good amount of thinking to uncover them.

The following attitudes are different ways of concealing fear:

Shyness. "I am embarrassed to express my opinion; they'll think I'm stupid or inadequate" means: I'm afraid to be misjudged in this situation.
Skepticism. "Why should I get involved? It's just politics" means: I'm afraid I'll be punished for my opinions if I commit myself.
Boredom. "Look, there's nothing out there; life is a drag" means: I'm afraid of assuming responsibility, or risking, or losing.
Hypocrisy. "Oh darling, I've missed you so much!" means: I'm afraid that if I don't say it, I won't be liked.

In general, we look at shyness, skepticism, boredom, and hypocrisy from different angles. For instance, we see shyness as a lack of self-confidence, skepticism as a philosophical posture, boredom as a lack of *joie de vivre,* and hypocrisy as an emotional lie. Although these interpretations are correct, it becomes important to dig out the root of the problem: fear.

Shyness, skepticism, boredom, and hypocrisy bear the characteristics of a cop-out system that builds itself into our personalities and becomes a pitiful representation of ourselves.

Understanding the cause of our fear will allow us to uncover its weak points. Knowing our fear's origin gives us the strength to fight back. The more knowledge we have about the fear, the better our self-confidence will be to counteract it. No matter what, let's face our fear. The worst thing to do is to deny it, because to live in fear will lead us to frustration, hatred, and anger.

Answer these questions before making any attempts to cope with fear:

1. What am I afraid of?
2. Do I understand the fear?
3. What are the disastrous consequences I will endure if I do nothing about it?
4. What will I gain if I do nothing about it?

Now we choose a method to get rid of fear. If we have been extensively damaged by fear, or we have become nonfunctional, or we suffer from serious anxiety or panic states, a professional consultation might be desirable. Treatment may include behavioral therapy, relaxation techniques, cognitive therapy, drug therapy, or a combination of any of these.

Self-help techniques should include (1) avoiding procrastination; (2) applying common sense to analyze fear; (3) developing self-confidence; and (4) gaining independence, thus assuming responsibility.

Fear is an unfair master to serve. It is used to control, achieve, hoard, and exploit. Remember, it is a minority that rules us all—a fearless minority.

Fear is provoked by those who control us all—the rulers of the world, the organized institutions that have amputated our freedom, those who speak of love while showing violence, the media when it lies, the society that scorns poetry and spiritual values, and those who judge but are corrupt. Do we accept slavery in order to survive? And if so, is mere survival enough?

At the Second Congress of the World Federation of Biological Psychiatry, I stated that the fear of losing one's mind is as grave as the fear of losing one's freedom. Because our imagination does not know of anatomical boundaries, it can fly away from bone and flesh. But if our mind becomes diseased, and no longer can fly, it remains imprisoned.

Sometimes I see myself running away for a self-encounter on a hypothetical summit. I am alone, naked, facing silence and open space, empty of fences, borders; my eyes taking me wherever I wish, listening to my heart pumping blood into my temples, recording the hissing of my breath, catching the air of nature with each hair of my body. I am ready to face myself with myself. But no one has ever taught me how to go about it. I do not like having to deal with myself, I am afraid to use my own judgment. I am afraid to confront my fears, my despair, my weakness. I don't want to accept myself as I am. I'd rather lie, obey the wrong command, condone corruption, worship alienation, accept bribes, defend my slaver, than confront my duties, my pride, my dreams, and my integrity. Will I be able to change?

To find oneself is to accept that one is alone from crib to grave. This loneliness means absolute freedom, and absolute freedom means absolute responsibility for ourselves, isolation from others, and acceptance of independence. To accept isolation in order to achieve freedom is a frightening proposition.

What a price to pay for freedom! What are the gains of becoming free if we must experience so much anguish? Are we saying that we live in fear if we are slaves, yet we also live in fear if we are free? Yes. But only up to a point. The lesson is that in slavery, we are *always* frightened, while in freedom, the fear is temporary, a transient presence during the process of becoming free.

Becoming free involves risking comfort, antagonizing people, challenging the immorality that pervades every layer of human relationships. Becoming free threatens our security, our jobs, our emotional lives, our privacy. Defiance toward slavery generates many kinds of fears, hesitations, and excuses. It brings frustration, embarrassment, and insomnia. The people closest to freedom have been the cowboy, the gaucho, and the nomad. Neither their land nor their courage was ever bounded by barbwire.

Freeing ourselves from fear should be a life priority. Unfortunately, the odds are against us. From babyhood on, our family, society, and government have been patiently teaching us how good it is not to be free. Therefore, we become frightened of the possibility! As a result, we use the easiest way out: slavery. Let the world be responsible for my welfare! I have no say in all this! Let my family, society, or government do it for me! A macho husband, an overworked wife, a puritanical society, and a tyrannical government are not impositions but choices made by fearful people.

Either we withdraw from the world or we remain in it. If we choose to remain as active members we will have to work very hard to undo our fears. Being frightened is the result of a lifelong process of conditioning.

We must develop mutual respect so love will replace violence and fear will assume a less important role in our lives. For if we don't develop respect, what hope do we hold for the future but the prospect of more violence, injustice, and corruption, and a supreme contempt for nature and human beings.

The epitaph of the Greek writer Nikos Kazantzakis says, "I want nothing, I fear nothing, I am free."

Anger

Are you telling me that I am an angry person because I yell, curse, and cut in front of cars that deserve to be taught a lesson? Are you suggesting that I am angry because when I wake up in the morning I refuse to interact in a civil manner? Do you feel I am angry because I slam doors, punch holes in walls, complain to clerks, waiters, and delivery boys? Because I am caustic with my parents, nasty to my children, scornful to you, mean to the poor, and cruel to strangers? Okay, I am angry! So what? When I feel angry, I do as I please. I don't feel I have to keep things inside.

Yes, I am angry. I have had it! Enough is enough! My wrath is the wrath of the just. I hate social injustice, my skin color does not match the required skin color so I hate it and I hate those who segregate me. Yes, I am angry because I don't have enough, because I am weak and I can't survive. I am angry when I cheat or when I am cheated. I am angry because I am not tall enough, bright enough or rich, beautiful, handsome, and powerful enough. But everyone is as angry as I am. Animals and plants, nature and the gods. Even newspapers say that if there are other worlds their inhabitants will be angry and hostile! So what's wrong if I'm angry? I couldn't care less whether you agree with me or not! People are angry, races are angry, countries, villages, and social clubs are angry! Who isn't angry? Only a jerk who meditates, writes poetry, and dreams of living in a hut in India wouldn't be angry! Don't you remember what Kazantzakis said in *The Greek Passion*? That Christ would come back with a can of oil to set the world on fire?!

Look at the leaders of the world, they are all angry. They want to reform the world on their own terms, for their own ambitions. Don't I have the lawful right to battle this world with all its contents? Violence is my best partner.

Sure thing, I am angry, and this is why.

Anger is caused by an unpleasant or frightening stimulus. When we are angry, our body muscles tense, our skin reddens, our heart beats faster, and our blood pressure rises. We are ready to curse, scream, break objects, assault, or kill.

In the brain, the centers of anger and fear are neighbors. We use anger to overcome fear. If we feel we are about to lose in a contest, fear and a desire to flee result. To remedy the situation, we stay and fight back—we show anger.

One factor leading to anger is frustration, the other, stress. Frustration is the feeling that follows an unfavorable outcome. Things often do not turn out the way we want—a job or a project falls through, a marriage fails. Stress disturbs the whole body, affecting our ability to remain calm. Under stress, nervousness and a tendency to react angrily are common.

From an angry thought to a violent action, anger carries different degrees of intensity. Whether we get visibly upset, enraged, or out of control, we need to develop coping mechanisms. Otherwise, angry behavior will become an outstanding feature of our personality. Physical anger is shown by assaulting others, hurting oneself, or breaking objects. Because of social pressures, physical anger is usually manifested at home. If we do not get rid of anger, it will get out in its own way. It may use the stomach, causing a peptic ulcer, or it may induce high blood pressure, a heart attack, a migraine, or depression.

Anger is a destructive force that threatens the foundations of the family and society. To the individual, anger brings social isolation, unhappiness, and increased frustration. To the integral being, or to those in the process of becoming one, anger is a serious handicap. Nonetheless, we may find positive aspects in our anger, if it gives rise to the mental and physical energy necessary to defend ourselves from acts of aggression. However, anger still ends up being a negative force.

Because anger is an emotion, we can't suppress it, but we can modify the behavior it sets off. We may still be angry inside, but we will be quiet on the outside if we take several deep breaths before we respond to aggression. Deep breathing, a relaxation exercise, works against the fast and shallow breathing that accompanies anger.

How do I recognize angry behavior? Is the anger reasonable or unreasonable? Common sense comes in handy here. Although identifying anger is certainly a priority, it sometimes is difficult to accomplish, especially for those who live in an angry environment. A hostile, competitive society, wars, police actions, and shoot-'em-up movies constitute an aggressive milieu. In a setting where violence is the norm, it becomes acceptable. Because people have a propensity to imitate others' behavior, these factors adversely affect our efforts for anger modification programs. If we live in this kind of environment, we should try to disconnect ourselves from it as much as we can.

A few years ago, a patient's wife called me in despair because her husband had destroyed the dining room table in a rage. Was this a first-time incident? I asked. Well, he used to beat her up, yell, and spank the children, but he never broke anything. She had accepted her husband's bad habits as normal. A broken piece of furniture was necessary to bring her husband's violence into focus.

Most of us have difficulty controlling our frustration. We feel the world owes us everything; we want it to go our way. Some of us have a need to dominate others—we are authoritarian, demanding, rigid. We measure world behavior by our own standards. We cannot tolerate imperfections, delays, indecisions, mediocrity, weaknesses. We forget that there is a limit to efficiency, and we should not set limits for the world. How many times do events or people's behaviors, even our own, fall short of our expectations? Expecting too much will fuel our anger. Tolerance is a great remedy for frustration.

Another way to modify anger is by asserting ourselves. When someone cuts in front of us in line to buy theater tickets, we have two choices—to show outward anger or to be assertive and politely ask the person to step aside. By using assertion we have more of a chance of getting what we want. An assertive person obtains more through firmly and fearlessly stating his or her feelings and desires.

Perhaps taking life less seriously would be the best medicine for anger. But if our aggression is out of control it is advisable to seek professional help.

Love

A friend told me that if I write on love I should avoid writing in a greeting card style. It is easy to fall into clichés with love, as so much has been written about it. I have decided, however, to take the risk of sounding like a greeting card, because the subject is a challenge. Besides, we should not confine love writing only to Valentine's Day.

A baby's mouth embracing a mother's nipple. Two hands clasped in a park. Young men saluting the flag, already veterans of war and suffering, experiencing gooseflesh for their country. The first moment of the first meeting between a woman and a man. The bereaved who still brings flowers to the cemetery. The idea of God and a solitary worshipper. A dog sitting by its master's chair. The lover poised to buy a single rose. The fast pumping of a heart, the racing of thoughts, the uncontrollable trembling of a first encounter. The sacrifice to work longer hours, the chunk of bread not eaten so the children can have it. The beautiful feeling that emanates from a deep region of the brain that, whether chemically or electrically programmed, forces us to stop our life for a second so we can feel, without reason, without calculation. Is it love?

In *Webster's* dictionary we find that love is "the attraction, desire, or affection felt for a person who arouses delight or admiration or elicits tenderness, sympathetic interest, or benevolence."

Although love is unidirectional, from the person who loves to the person being loved, it requires reciprocity. To love without being loved is painful and absurd.

For me, love is a strong attraction to someone who elicits the need to care, to possess and be possessed, and the urge to be told that I exist and I am unique. When we find love, then we share. As the poet Kahlil Gibran once wrote, "Fill each other's cup but drink not from one cup."

Although love is an emotion to be exchanged between people, its application has encompassed other objects of love. There is social love, which involves love for our work or job, animals, nature, cities, and countries. There is philosophical love, which interacts with religion, philosophy, and the universe in general.

Certain forms of love go beyond our physical world, questioning the premise that only people can be loved. Some religions have chosen higher levels of loving experience known as mysticism. For those who practice it, mysticism is extraordinarily rewarding. Al-Hallach, the ninth-century Arab mystic, wrote, "I am the One I love, and That One that I love is MYSELF—we are two spirits coming to dwell in a single body."

Love, like any other emotion, is within ourselves, ready to be awakened. We don't have to learn how to fall in love, and we know when it happens, from mental and physical responses. All of a sudden another person is at the center of our thoughts; we feel good, happy, daring. Our skin gets gooseflesh, the heart pumps faster, the blood pressure goes up, energy flows in a continuous gallop, the need to eat or sleep is reduced. Our attention and all of our senses are shut off from the rest of the world.

Love lasts as long as our interest in its object remains alive. Conversely, it is the obligation of the object to keep us interested because love, like any other emotion, is a response to a stimulus. Love is an emotion of attraction, the way fear is an emotion of retraction, and anger an emotion of repulsion. Hence, love, as an attracter, binds the world together.

Love summons up a constellation of different emotions.

When we are in love we care, we doubt, we are jealous, possessive, sexual, ambitious; we feel like a god being worshipped or like a slave following a master. Love is the realization that perhaps we are not alone, that we need others. The idea that we long for someone, that we cannot live as loners shakes our individuality and our freedom. For most people, to fall in love and form a lasting relationship is one of the main goals in life. Of course, falling in love does not always lead to a lasting relationship, and sometimes we are merely infatuated. Infatuation is a strong but unreasonable attraction to a person, a transient form of love.

Love can also be disrupted by the presence of jealousy. This emotion questions the honesty and behavior of our beloved one. It reflects a need to possess and not share the object of our love with others. When intense, jealousy assumes pathological consequences—remember Othello and his misguided distrust of Desdemona.

Jealousy implies several behaviors. The lover who begs to be loved and has to be continuously reassured of being loved. The lover who demands total submission of the beloved, interfering with his or her social and working activities, or banning them altogether. The lover who is highly critical and mercilessly accuses the loved one for just about everything. The lover who demands love and, if not granted, goes through incredible self-punitive behavior, not eating, becoming depressed, refusing to work or to leave the house. And there is the jealous lover who is vengeful and reacts by dating others, bringing additional distress to the relationship.

The integral being reacts toward jealousy with understanding and tolerance. If doubts about fidelity arise, dialogue is the answer. The integral being knows that true trust and dialogue are essential.

To love and be loved is the most important aid to becoming an integral person. Love gives an opportunity to care and to share, to know and to respect. To be loved offers us recognition of our individuality, support for our struggle, care for our needs, and tenderness for our moments of dependency.

For the integral being, love is an emotion with social repercussions. Love could make the individual and society share possessions. But because sharing goes against profit making and greed, love is discouraged. Love is only profitable in economic terms, when we buy a diamond to show it. On the other hand, violence promotes sales. What is the price of a kiss or a hug against the price of a cruise missile?

The continuous invasion of ruthless materialism systematically destroys our freedom to love. Human actions are becoming more and more influenced by mechanization. In order to control human behavior, there is a trend to suppress love and promote two emotions in its stead: anger and fear. On an individual basis, self-centered egotistical life-styles demand narcissistic love. As this is in opposition to social love, we see the same consequence of love in decline.

I am afraid that love is dying. Is it that love stimuli are lacking? In a world ruled by fear and anger, love looks like a war refugee—hungry, lost, and resentful.

In some cultures, love seems to be relegated to movies or books, disregarding individual manifestations. To show love is embarrassing, a symbol of weakness or subservient behavior. Kissing, embracing, holding hands, even handshaking are becoming obsolete in certain cultures. Most of these physical contacts appear to be accepted only in the context of lovemaking. We keep saying, "Let's keep in touch." But how? The only touching I can think of is when traveling on overcrowded buses.

Love should help us to fulfill our needs on earth, to share what we are and what we have, to care for others, and to be taken care of. In love, we have to be truthful and faithful. We must understand the feelings and needs of the person we love. We have to show support and encouragement during difficult times. Above all, we have to respect the beloved. Only mutual respect will preserve love as it should be: a source of life energy and hope enabling us to endure our time on this earth.

Duty

At the beginning of my life I was told not to touch this and that; a year later, though my walking was the cause for celebration, my boundaries were restricted by gates, balconies, screens, and so forth. Eventually I was forced to spoon-feed myself. By the age of four—already toilet-trained—it was suggested I should only touch my penis for the sole purpose of urination. Prayers became a daily routine to save me from hell. In school I learned I should not lie and that I had to obey my teachers. When I began to attend mass I found out I was a sinner. During my adolescence I learned that my rebelliousness could kill my father with a heart attack. At the age of eighteen, I learned I should be proud of my forceful enlistment in the army. You have duties and sacrifices for your motherland. Don't make love, the lure of flesh will destroy your future. You should be a doctor. Respect your elders, be fair to your friends. Get married, have children, support a family, take care of your patients, be faithful, don't make a business out of your life, pay your taxes, drive carefully, be successful, watch your cholesterol, abhor red meat, and take vitamins.

One day I envision myself electronically plugged into this world and people telling me, "You must not die, your duty is to remain alive."

Ask for three important human traits and I will mention laziness, innocence, and fearfulness. To prove my point, I lie down underneath a shady tree on a summer afternoon adopting a Huckleberry Finn attitude toward the world. Suddenly, someone gently taps me on the shoulder to bring me back from my dream world, demanding that I go back to school. How did they know I was here? I have failed my *duty* and I feel guilty.

Belief, faith, and duty guide our behavior. I know that belief is what I accept as true, and I agree with Nietzsche that faith is not wanting to know what is true. But when it comes to duty, I have more difficulty accepting it because of the multiplicity of elements that compose what we feel and know as duty.

Duty is a social emotion that compels us to act in a certain way to fulfill our moral and legal obligations. Duty is second to love in the psychological makeup of the integral being. To have a solid and powerful sense of duty does wonders to achieve integration. An integral being operates within the societal structure abiding by the law and performing tasks oriented to the care of others.

The ancients did not have many duties toward others because they lived in secluded small groups. The growth of the human race created a supersocial being who in modern life is continuously burdened by obligations. These obligations are the result of knowing what is right and what is wrong. We all live by a value system that includes our personal moral code and the code of the society we live in. This value system is controlled by our judgment, which approves or disapproves our feelings, thoughts, and behavior.

Without a sense of duty, we cannot live in society. Family, society, and government are very demanding. It is difficult to conceive of a society without a minimum set of established rules and regulations. Without these, a society would perish in chaos.

In order to establish a sense of duty we are taught the word *must,* which connotes obligation, requirement, indispensability, and other meanings related to duty. The concept of *must* is learned through education and social interaction. Toilet training is an early must. Later we learn to say: I must work, I must provide, I must pay my taxes, and so on. Must is activated by conviction—we believe we are doing the right thing; and by fear—we don't believe we are doing the right thing, but we are afraid of being punished or having to live with our guilt.

Because we are creatures of moral habits, a code of rules known as law gradually evolved. The law determines what is right and wrong for us and punishes us if we break the rules. Our own law should be the same as the social law, otherwise we become outlaws. To avoid trouble, we have developed a set of behavioral responses known as obedience.

To obey others is to submit oneself to the will of third parties who may or may not agree with our wishes. Although obedience might be at times a disappointing response, it has its advantages. For example, obedience reduces individual responsibility for our actions. If anything goes wrong, we simply blame it on those who commanded the action. This loss of individual responsibility is seen in every huge government or commercial institution where anonymity and following orders are the rule.

Obedience for the sake of obedience, or "blind obedience," may challenge our personal value systems. A soldier dies on the battlefield in defiance of his instinct for survival or the moral code that forbids killing. Duty is an emotion that can go against our vital needs.

Nowadays, young people do not have many "dutiful heroes" to emulate. If they do, those heroes are usually scorned by a social system fed with the cynical doctrine that proposes deceit as the means to achieve success and fame. The answer is to remind families, societies, and governments that they all have laws and duties to abide by. However, there are often two sets of laws, one for private and one for public consumption:

1. A parent who says, "Do not smoke marijuana" but has three martinis before dinner.
2. A society that preaches equal rights but practices segregation.
3. A government that declares justice for all yet has more laws to limit freedom than to give freedom.
4. A religion that bans abortion in order to preserve life but tolerates wars.
5. A legal system designed to provide justice for all, but because of court costs favors only those in the high income brackets.

Duty draws justice into the social arena. Law links justice and duty. The three complement each other; if they don't, generalized injustice results. We begin to question whether we are engaged in sheer stupidity by playing the role of the altruist. A continuous display of injustice challenges our integrity and results in the alienation of individuals, families, societies, and nations. We resort to semantics: what used to be unjust is now just, and vice versa.

An integral being is a duty-bound person with a high degree of responsibility. An integral being finds satisfaction and joy in accomplishment, reinforcing the disposition to perform and deliver. An integral being is dutiful by conviction, not by imposition. The sense of obligation is the result of reasoning and love. An integral being is cognizant of the roughness of human interaction and knows that mutual respect smooths the way. Without mutual respect, duty as a social emotion is difficult to accept, inasmuch as a given duty may affect our own welfare.

Because integral beings are efficient and prompt to oblige, they might be burdened by an excess of obligations. People quickly identify and single out these individuals and overwhelm them with tasks. But we should not live for others twenty-four hours a day. Sometimes others will have to help ease our life. We must remember we all have to participate and share. An excessive load of duties can affect our health. We must grow as trees do in the forest—in spite of crowding, they search for the sun.

Duty reminds me of a graffiti written on the wall of the airport of a totalitarian country that said, "The last one to leave, please switch off the lights."

Envy

In 1665, La Rochefoucauld wrote in *Maxims,* "Our envy always lasts much longer than the happiness of those we envy." We all know the painful desire to have what others have. To have sharp brains, beautiful bodies, a house with an indoor swimming pool, a luxurious car, social status, children in Ivy League schools, a brilliant marriage. Envy is an emotion that makes us uncomfortably aware of advantages others have over us. We don't discuss our envy with others because envy is a socially unacceptable emotion. Envious people use subterfuge and seductive behavior to obtain what they want; to avoid social criticism, they operate behind the scenes.

Envy develops as the result of unreasonable desires to own and to have. Because envy is an emotion, we have to expect to feel envious here and there. But allowing envy to become a dominant emotion means trouble.

Is envy a shameful emotion? Is envy sinful? Is envy an illness? My answer to all three is yes. Yet, in all my years of psychiatric practice, I have never seen a patient walk into my office to get rid of envy, although it will slowly destroy our happiness, and, surely, our growth as integral beings.

To envy we go through a process of comparisons. What we have versus what they have, what our advantages are versus theirs. Usually we end up feeling we have less, dissatisfied with our findings, and resentful. From then on, envy entwines with greed, a growing selfishness, and a loss of joy in our lives.

Envious people are ignorant of their resources and demand or expect to get beyond the reach of the possibilities. Typically, those who envy lack self-limits; they overvalue their own skills, and hence become frustrated (and frustration leads to anger, with all its consequences).

An envious person cannot be generous, inasmuch as possessions offer security and a sense of self-realization. The behavior of the envious person is conducive to isolation within the family and the social circle. When envy is a secret emotion, however, it may be difficult to identify.

We should check for envy if we find ourselves wishing to

have more than others; if we manifest feelings that the world owes us everything; if we feel distressed, angry, or unhappy after learning about someone's achievement; if we become extremely critical of others; or if we are intolerant of other people or other environments. With any of these, envy may be creeping up on us.

"Keeping up with the Joneses" is the neighborhood malady of competing for achievement and material ownership. What appears to be a highly recommended endeavour at first glance is just an illogical race in which the participants exhaust themselves, usually beyond their aptitudes.

What do we do to correct envy? One way is to control our indiscriminate need to have. Society, working through the mass media, would persuade us that to be consumers is a cherished goal in life. Toward that purpose, advertisements lure us to buy, regardless of our needs or buying power.

In popular magazines and on television shows the lives of celebrities are praised, inflated, and worshipped. It is disgraceful that we are invited to live vicariously through the lives of those we envy. With envy, we come to identify with our idol, and eventually we "own" the worshipped object: "*My* hero." This sort of vicarious existence conceals our reality and postpones our achievements, relegating us to the roles of spectators of life.

If we really want to have the prestige, the wealth, the health, or the love that others have, we must work for it. Sitting in front of a television screen feeling sorry for ourselves will not help.

Suppose you are stricken by an urge to have and you decide to do something constructive with your envy. You honestly ask yourself what you want from life. Set goals that are reasonable and within your reach. Assess your limitations. Then, you are ready to go out and get it. This is a process of emulation, not of envy, and it usually works.

When we become integral, envy is automatically discarded. Other emotions dominate our lives, like love and duty. We can never be certain, however, that envy will not show up. But self-introspection and analyzing our behavior, desires, and dreams will provide us with enough clues to detect any upsurge of envious feelings. Let us bring our own pride into the light. Let us be proud of who we are and what we have. Chances are that frustration will ensue, until we get used to living with less.

Two other factors used to curtail envy are self-discipline and sacrifice. If we are too much creatures of comfort, we jeopardize our goal to become integral. It is important to learn how to do without. One technique to test our capacity for sacrifice and discipline is to fast. To do without food postpones gratification, builds up willpower, and temporarily removes us from other matters. Fasting (under control) is practical for those who want to develop spiritually.

Avarice

One day I took a smooth pebble in my hand and, for a moment, I thought that I held the universe in that small, perfect stone. Years later, life showed me how wrong I was.

We are animals of endless needs, among them, the need to possess. We call this avarice, although all it is is greed dressed up with a fancy name.

From time immemorial we have counted—with the calendar, bones, money, people, cattle. There is a census for everything. A human being owns, collects, stores, saves, hoards. Counting is a way of knowing how much we have, in order to monitor growth or loss. The counting of the avaricious differs in that they count only to add, never to subtract. When the old lady down the block died, the neighbors collected money to give her a decent funeral. They were shocked when they found her mattress stuffed with one-hundred-dollar bills and passbooks for savings accounts, worth enough to cover the cost of several funerals.

Greedy people usually live below their economic means. To accumulate without enjoyment is an outstanding characteristic of avarice. The outcome is a life of deprivation. The house becomes a huge attic for unused objects and money. For others, avarice is a need to accumulate food, clothing, jewelry, or books in excess of need.

As human beings we are faced with the dilemma of having to choose what is good for us. Current trends indicate that what is good for the system we live in is what counts. Society comes before our personal welfare.

So far, the majority has chosen to imitate the rich minority. Power and money are sought after by millions of people; most of them die in their pursuit without reaching their goals. Few choose a more sensible, compromising goal to limit their aspirations to more realistic aims. Others have plainly rejected materialism, choosing to follow the path of the great masters of religion who preached austerity.

It was about two o'clock in the morning when the emergency call came in. It took ten minutes for the ambulance to get there. She was seventeen years old when she decided to put a shotgun in her mouth and blow her head apart. She lay in the living room, surrounded by police and expensive furniture. Her mother was crying. "My daughter had maids, cars, beauty, and intelligence. Why did she kill herself?" the mother asked tearfully. I still wonder if that young girl had love, hope, innocence, or a family to speak of. Such a sad end exemplifies the loss of equilibrium between possession and moral and spiritual values.

Either we are, and feel, or we have. In other words, to be or to have.

Do we want to have because others have? The learning process of having begins at birth. This is your food, this is your toy, this is your room, this is your chair. I have parents, he is my doctor, this is my country, I have children, I own a house, I have money in the bank. We are taught that wealth provides freedom of will and movement; we find out that money buys material things. Our society worships material things as symbols of success and independence. In those parts of the world geared to consumerism we can observe the disastrous consequence of a materialistic society in the breakdown of the moral foundations of the country.

We are gigantic mouths with bottomless guts. I was shocked when, on my arrival in the United States, I was asked how much my father was worth. The question was stupifyingly beyond my comprehension.

We want to be integral beings but we have developed avarice. What can we do about it?

The process of accumulation requires time—to obtain, to preserve, and to increase the number of our possessions. This time is diverted from the time we need to take care of ourselves. As integral beings we need time to take care of our bodies, emotional and intellectual needs. We cannot live in a continuously acquisitive state. A more contemplative state will allow us to develop as integrals. Contemplation opens the gates to higher levels of consciousness, bringing insight into ourselves and feelings of peace and self-contentment. These new attitudes will help us to dispose of worldly possessions we deem excessive or unnecessary.

• • • *Chapter Eight*

THE INTELLECT

> The man who listens to Reason is lost: Reason enslaves all whose minds are not strong enough to master her.
>
> George Bernard Shaw, *Man and Superman* (1903)

If we decide to quit work, drop out of school, neglect our health, or procrastinate, we lack willpower. If we leave our body at the mercy of the tempestuous forces of our emotions, or if we decide to live by instinct, we are lost. To avoid these things, we have a mind, or intellect.

The intellect controls the power to feel and to will, so we can live with ourselves and others in harmony. Hence, the intellect is the pivotal force in the making of the integral being.

As the philosophical seat of our brain, the intellect is instrumental in queries about our origin. Intellectual activity is highly driven by curiosity. Why? how? what? when? where? compose the basic vocabulary of the intellect. The mind is interested in facts, fantasies, beliefs, and ideas. The mind explores, observes, registers, analyzes, judges, decides, executes, and does. If properly trained, the mind may even modify certain physiological activities, such as reducing blood pressure through biofeedback or meditation techniques.

The intellect is the greatest coordinator of our lives, a tireless policymaker constantly looking after our welfare. Without our intellect, it would be impossible to live the way we do. Technological advancement, the conquering of disease, space travel, art, music, and literary masterpieces exist as proof of our intellectual performance. Furthermore, intellectual activities are not hindered by the boundaries of our senses. With our imagination, we can fly high and to faraway places. We can move into unexplored regions of the mind and establish contact with the world at a higher level of consciousness.

In order to become integral beings, we must write a program tailored to our needs, which considers our handicaps. Ortega y Gasset, the Spanish philosopher, said, "Man invents himself a program of life to answer the difficulties imposed by circumstances."

To make a program, we must get acquainted with ourselves, just as we did with our body and emotions, but in this case, with our intellect.

The first question we ask is, Who am I?

We are told we are essence, a common denominator for all living matter, a human body.

We are told we are existence, alive, but as one unit with a distinct face and a name.

We are told we are presence, we occupy a physical space.

We are told we are what we do, our trade modifies who we are.

So we are essence, existence, presence, and actions.

We get acquainted with our intellect as we do with our body. A mirror will not reflect our brain, however, nor a stethoscope detect an intellectual thump. But when we explore a forest and discover a new plant, or when we judge someone's behavior, or when we play a musical instrument, remember past episodes of our life, build a house, or write a poem, we are in touch with our intellect.

There are several intellectual activities; to observe, to think, to execute, to make, and to create. These are irreplaceable functions meant to enhance our well-being, and we should use them accordingly.

The observer registers the events, the thinker analyzes them, the executor carries the answer, the maker performs the task, and the creator rejects accepted logic and moves a step forward.

The Observer

One day, in our mother's womb, we paid attention to her heartbeat and to the liquid in which we floated. We felt warm, safe, at peace. At that point we became the observer. Observers carry the curiosity that takes us through life. Our curiosity is inexhaustible because every new day new stimuli are brought to our attention. Late in life, after thousands of sensorial experiences, our curiosity diminishes, and we become more introspective. By keeping ourselves curious enough throughout life, we will slow our aging process, because curiosity brings enthusiasm, surprise, and the joy to make each day a new one.

Our brain is continuously bombarded with thousands of stimuli. Strolling down a street, we are receptors for the sounds and movement of cars and people, the colors of clothing and neon signs, the smell of the street vendor's food, and the music of a record shop. Suddenly, behind our backs we hear a noise. Someone drops a bag and a bottle breaks. Of all the stimuli that we were receiving in our brain, we selected this one. We paid attention to it.

Attention is the condition in which we focus upon one stimulus out of thousands. We pay attention to the size of the stimulus—a skyscraper that surpasses others. We also pay attention to the noise of a stimulus—a thunderbolt heard above the sound of rain. Attention is also influenced by our personal interests or motivations. For instance, we pay attention to an interesting conversation or a movie character with whom we identify. We also pay attention to repetitive stimuli, such as, in the silence of the night, the sound of dripping water in the bathroom. Our body also produces stimuli that cause us to pay attention: a tight collar, new shoes that squeeze our feet, an aching tooth.

Why is it important to pay attention? On one level, it is for the purpose of survival; on another level, it is for the purpose of learning. The integral being develops this faculty with care, because attention is the first step in integrating knowledge. A well-trained, observing mind will result in a better analytical mind. The whole process of learning can be disrupted by a short attention span.

Learning involves comprehension, analysis, discrimination, reasoning, comparison, and memory. We go about learning in passive and active ways. The passive system is reading, listening, seeing; the active system is experimental. The main sources of learning are schools, books, the media, the street, other people, and personal experience.

Schools are by far the leading center of education. The ideal educational system should be free. Moreover, it should be a system where the educational material is unbiased in reference to civic subjects and history. But more important, schools are meant to teach the people how to read and write.

A book establishes an extraordinary rapport between the reader and the writer, between the observer and the stimulus. For an integral being, books are an important source of information during the formative years. By choosing our reading material, we establish a degree of independence. In addition, for those unable or unwilling to complete higher levels of education, books are great teachers. Many great men and women are self-taught.

Media adds a new dimension to education by making it accessible to a broad audience. Because modern media has surpassed geographical borders, it might be used to exchange national programs geared to improve international understanding and acceptance of different sociopolitical systems. In remote areas, television brings teaching programs otherwise unavailable.

The street is probably the oldest teacher on earth. Any "pushcart" millionaire knows that well. Relatives, friends, and parents offer us their behaviors, examples, and experience as another way of learning. Finally, the great educator of experience becomes enriched by age and also by a life intense with action and commitment.

And what do we learn? First of all, we learn about us—our physical and mental makeup, our emotions, our intellect. Then we learn about the systems we live in—family, society, government, and nature. In addition to learning a trade, we learn about human interactions, social norms and customs, and the functions and purposes of things. We learn what is applicable to our own interests.

At this point, we begin to correlate. We look for associations, connections, interdependencies. We unfold mechanisms of coexistence so we can understand the need to integrate in order to harmonize.

By the process of learning we integrate ourselves, and we gradually incorporate ourselves in the world mechanism, not as an isolated part of the world but as the whole itself. By learning, we actively engage ourselves in life affairs, and our whole selves will automatically move into a new dimension of perception, understanding, and enjoyment.

A reminder: Always be alert in order to learn.

The process of observing and attending to is complemented by the process by which information is retained. This keeper is our memory, which stores and retrieves every single event we have experienced since we were born. Once we have observed, we convert that material to chemical compounds which are then stored in several areas of our brain. If we ever need to retrieve this material, a chemical messenger makes the delivery. We can store material for a few seconds or many years.

It has been suggested that some memory material can be passed on in our genes from generation to generation. In 1962, J. V. McConnell trained planarians, a type of worm, with certain forms of conditioning. Then these planarians were ground up and fed to other planarians. The new planarians were more rapidly conditioned than those who were not fed their predecessors. Further studies with higher forms of life, such as rats and fishes, confirmed the chemical theory of the transfer of memory.

Although many memory studies are controversial, their findings are important and encouraging. Is memory found in instinct? Did our ancestors learn things that we now know without having to study? Many mysteries remain to be unraveled.

In this regard, Carl Jung, the Swiss psychiatrist, spoke of a collective unconscious, or collective memory. While I was doing my medical internship in Buenos Aires, a twelve-year-old girl was admitted to the emergency room. She was in a trance, talked to herself, and was extremely agitated. But in her delirium she only spoke English. According to her mother, the girl had never learned English, her ancestors were all Spanish. Hours later, the girl recovered with no recollection of the happening.

Was my patient a recipient of someone else's memory? Would a collective memory influence our integral development? In time, we hope to explain these mysteries.

Intellectual functions have to be looked after with adequate care. It is known that our brain cortex completes its development after our birth. During this postnatal period our brain anatomy can grow bigger if enough stimulation and information are provided. Scientists have shown that rats kept solitary or with few objects around developed less brain weight than rats raised in an enriched environment. Moreover, information is stored in protein, which is derived from what we eat. We must have both food and information to develop a normal brain.

Famine and illiteracy, present in many regions of the world, are already breeding a race of underdeveloped brains that will be useful as cheap slave labor. What better way to control people than to deprive the young of food and information? We may further question the information provided to our young by the mass media. Will it alter the growth of their intellectual and emotional functions? Frightening, isn't it? But it is already happening.

Accepting that memory is a fundamental piece of the intellectual mechanism, it is essential to preserve it. Many people complain of memory loss. Most of the time, it is caused by lack of attention. This is the case of anxious individuals or hyperactive children, who have very short attention spans. Other times, people subconsciously choose to forget unpleasant events; they learn to block and deny past situations. In the elderly, memory loss is sometimes present due to hardening of brain arteries or as the result of brain atrophy, such as Alzheimer's disease. Memory loss can also be seen in older people taking medications that adversely affect brain functioning.

What do we do to keep our memory in shape? Usually, nothing, because we take for granted that our memory is good and will always be that way. In general, this is true; our memory services itself. However, memory can be improved, developed, and—what is more important—preserved. We know that there is not yet a good tonic for the memory, but there are exercises. The best ones are to remember poetry, historical dates, and facts.

The Thinker

If we decide not just to observe our life, we will have to think about it. We will become thinkers.

We think with the lateral parts of our brain. These areas are connected to the rest of the brain by several anatomical and electrochemical circuits, so thought messages can travel from place to place. To think, we use words, images, and melodies. Thinking is also facilitated by our muscles and vocal chords. Muscles move very subtly when we think, and vocal chords move, too, as if we were speaking out loud. This mind-muscle connection is representative of the mental and motor integration of our body.

When we are faced with a problem we gather information and proceed to think in progressive stages of analysis, comparison, association, discrimination, and choice. The capacity for efficient thinking and the ability to process information with accuracy and speed is called intelligence.

An intelligent thinker uses other resources than the known mental functions to think. As integral beings, we gather all our experience and knowledge to face a problem, analyzing matters with a subjective and objective lens. Is the problem a technical, emotional, moral, or social issue? Accordingly we will apply a quota of pragmatism, passion, compassion, and fairness. Only then will we make a decision and act upon it.

Most of us do not have time to think. We are living in an era of speed in technology, life-styles, and even emotional involvements. Lack of time, rushing in and out of situations, weakens the power of thinking. Quick thinking is not necessarily an indication of intelligent thinking. Lack of time can interfere with our capacity to screen information before storing it; we need to separate correct from incorrect information and truth from lies. If we continuously store erroneous information, we will operate erroneously when we retrieve it. Because we are living in a world where lies and deceit are common we will think and behave with confusion.

As a consequence of the continuous input of information we become stressed, intolerant, and impulsive. Many people react to stress situations with impulsive responses. When we do this, the gains are minimal because an impulse carries little thinking but a great instinctual and emotional load that is often wrong.

Frequently we replace thinking by employing previously learned mechanisms of response. We operate automatically with behavior that has been reinforced by our daily routines. In this fashion, we perform our daily chores, but presented with a serious matter or an emotional issue to solve, we will have to think.

Due to technological advancements, our thinking has also been partly replaced by computers and mass media, which deliver predigested information.

As a consequence of these modern trends in the thinking process, our brains have become lazy. We are losing the ability to think abstractly. However, there is not much stimulation for serious thinking in a society that favors light topics, banal books, and shallow films. Without an evolving, thinking brain, as individuals or as a social group, we will regress as human beings.

Unfortunately none of us is immune to the hazards of mental disorders affecting our thinking process. We have to preserve our capacity to think and, most important, do our own thinking. A homemade thought is better than a borrowed one. We should not mortgage our freedom of thought.

The Executor

We digest our observations by analyzing, comparing, classifying, and associating stimuli, then ordering our ideas. We register in memory what we have learned, so we may recall the information if need be. After that we are ready to respond to the stimulus. We know that every person has different reactions to a stimulus; this is our individuality. We also know that every stimulus demands a response. Therefore we elaborate on an idea or a set of concepts in our mind. We then have to choose how to act. This is known as decision making. Then we are ready to execute the order.

There are several factors in decision making. First, our

ability to choose, which is based on our judgment. The quality of our ability to choose determines not only the degree of involvement in our life, but our decision to become an integral being or not. We have the choice to be or not, to do or not, to live or not. Second, decision making requires certainty to make the decision, responsibility to act upon it, and willpower to implement the order.

Three saboteurs prowl the territory of decision making: doubt, fear, and procrastination. As soon as we lower our defenses we are invaded by hesitation, fear of making the wrong decision, or an unavoidable urge to postpone it. Thus programs, proposals, jobs, marriages—in general, our capacity to perform—are jeopardized.

If we cannot make decisions as the result of an emotional disorder, low self-esteem, self-destructive behavior, depression, or dependency, we must correct these conditions. Our whole program to become an integral will stall if we cannot decide. There is no magic formula to make the right decision, but there are a few steps that can help. One is to develop our self-esteem, stop overanalyzing, and be assertive. Another, the most important aid for decision making, is to use common sense, that "sense" we rarely employ. Finally, to be aware that our decision may upset others who will criticize or turn against us. We must remain independent and not be afraid of failing.

The outcome of decision making is called judgment. The better the decisions we make, the better the judgment we have. Judgment can be easily impaired when mixed with emotion. When decisions are related to interpersonal problems, emotional pros and cons are always present, which can weaken our capacity to judge.

Utilitarian persons will be devoid of emotion when making a decision, whereas self-expressionists will use emotion.

The integral being will look for harmony between judgment and emotion and enough time to think and feel before making a decision. Let us remember that when thinking takes over emotion, freedom moves rapidly away.

We are habits and passions, circumstances of life, milestones in history. As a race we are strikingly similar, and as individuals we are fundamentally different. We make the decision to blend ourselves with earth as we grow and mature.

After much reading, thinking, feeling, and discussing I came to the understanding in my life that either I changed on my own terms and of my own volition or I was going to stagnate. There was no time to regret past error or to start all over again. I refused to fool myself and keep postponing my changes. I said to myself: Perhaps new generations will uncover the secret of making a more humanistic history. The one we have, the one our ancestors left to us, is simply deplorable. I made the important decision to become an integral being. And I had a very powerful motivation: a strong desire to remain healthy and free.

The Maker

Reason distinguishes us from other animals. But all our power to think, decide, and execute would be fruitless had we not hands to make it visible. Archeologists have identified the first time we used our hands as instruments of our brain in Kenya, where they found the first chopping tools. They were 2,600,000 years old.

We are toolmakers who over the centuries have perfected our craft. We have made tools to build houses, instruments to play music, and weapons to kill. We are restless architects who have always had an extraordinary desire to build big—the Great Wall of China, the pyramids of Egypt. Once our decision is made, we do.

Why do we work so hard? We work for survival, for trade, for pleasure, for sheer pride. Our social customs expect us to work, our government obliges us to work, and our family demands it.

Some people feel compelled to work, an irresistible force to do things. They are known as compulsive workers. Compulsive workers have a utilitarian, with puritanical overtones, view of life. They have no time for pleasure except that experienced by the actual process of work, not the pleasure felt with the finished product. A long-term achiever, the compulsive worker runs the world we live in.

The amount of work we perform is determined by our attitude toward it, our needs, ambition, or obligations. From the social perspective, work availability is determined by the needs of the market. Without jobs, we are subject to the whims of charitable institutions or welfare. A well-developed society is one without unemployment.

But do we have to work?

We left Paradise long ago. Our reality tells us that we must be breadwinners but the idea of *a dolce far niente* ("it's sweet to do nothing") is tempting. We are basically playful animals, and, given the opportunity, we are usually ready to stop working and enjoy other things in life. A touch of hedonism is desirable. Although work might be a gratifying activity, most of it is routine.

To answer our inner wishes for a long-lasting vacation, we now have robots that can make decisions, fly planes, build automobiles, and solve problems. The word *robot* is derived from the Czech word *robota*, meaning "forced labor." This word was coined by the Czech playwright Karel Capek in his play *Rossun's Universal Robots*. A robot today may take the place of a worker and thus become part of the labor force, but do not fear: the toolmaker still builds the robots.

How important is the maker in the process of becoming an integral being?

The whole idea of the maker, or doer, is to perform, to materialize concepts. Doing is equal to action. The process of becoming an integral being requires doing. An integral being is also a doer, because one aspect of our reason to be is to do, and we are what we do. To maintain nature, we must perform.

The integral being is equipped with the instruments to perform. We have the capacity to build and to destroy, two forces also found in nature, where the elements are balanced by biology and ecology. But human beings employ feelings as determinants to build or destroy. When negative feelings predominate we tend to destroy.

Certainly we build to destroy. But we should only destroy what is decayed or obsolete. The kind of destruction to avoid is war and moral annihilation. It is the duty of the integral being to build, preserve, and defend our world.

Humans are blessed and cursed by becoming the maker. The rapid industrialization and technological advances of the world are mind-boggling. Because we did not grow in harmony with the universe, we forgot that life must be integral within nature.

We are a species full of contradictions. Human beings are more altruistic, bizarre, unpredictable, erratic, and violent than the entire universe; it is more difficult to explain a human being than to explain the orbiting of the planets. We need to learn the laws of equilibrium from the universe. We act with determination because we feel alive without fear, we feel we know ourselves inside and out. We are observers, thinkers, executors, and makers. And, no matter what our circumstances, we will still have the ability to create.

The Creator

Once upon a time an apple, the fruit of wisdom and temptation, fell on the head of Isaac Newton, and gravity, the element that nails us to earth, became known. Until then, how many people had an apple fall on their head? Yet none came up with a theory of gravitational force. Newton made sense of two things that appeared to be unrelated, an apple and its fall, and obtained something new. Newton was a creator.

In every brain there is a sector for creativity just waiting to be used. Our brain has learned to distinguish what is helpful from what is harmful. We want to be safe, so we use our instincts and reflexes to protect ourselves from an environment that can be hostile. To control this environment, we become creators.

Symbols, logic, daydreaming, imagination are some of the tools that creators use to perform their craft. The main characteristic of creative people is their originality. Creators are usually obsessed with their ideas and become compulsive workers, but at times they stop completely until new inspiration arrives. Creators hardly ever conform to the existing order. They are individualists who cheer freedom and resist established traditions and authority. Some creators are self-centered, living in their own worlds. Others are socially oriented. Some will show a well-developed aesthetic sense, others will not. Although overall their personalities are not always the same, creators have a tendency to be anxious. Their moods may fluctuate without apparent reason.

We usually associate creativity with the arts and the sciences. However, not every composer, poet, painter, scientist, philosopher, craftsperson, or social reformer is a creator. Ordinarily, we are imitators or followers. Most times, poets and musicians merely rearrange the order of words, meanings, and sounds. Occasionally, poets and musicians introduce new creations. We have old and we have new creations. We keep reinventing the past.

Am I saying that few of us are true creators? Exactly, although I believe we all have the components to give birth to a creation. For this we need time to observe and think. We must not be overly preoccupied with our daily routines, we must not fear becoming independent. These attitudes will discourage any creative potential that we may harbor within ourselves. We have to be free to create.

Does an integral being need to be a creator? No. Creativity is a faculty that will not assist us in our search for health, freedom, and knowledge. However, if we use the word *creator* as a synonym for *innovation,* if we call the result of making ourselves integral beings an act of creation, then we can be creators. If we consider our presence on this earth as an absurd or senseless episode, if we see ourselves as nonsensical beings, this is our chance to make sense of what seems to be senseless—a truly creative act.

··· Chapter Nine

ON DISEASE

> Between the desire
> And the spasm
> Between the potency
> And the existence
> Between the essence
> And the descent
> Falls the Shadow.
>
> T. S. Eliot,
> "The Hollow Men" (1925)

The nineteenth-century French scientist Claude Bernard posited the theory that the body has the capacity to maintain equilibrium within itself and within the surrounding biological environment. He called this function *milieu intérieur,* or homeostasis.

A disease is the loss of equilibrium within ourselves or between ourselves and our external environment. This equilibrium has to be extended to the sociopolitical environment because we may also acquire disease through contamination with a diseased society.

We are like a triangle—the three sides are body, emotions, and intellect—and we must maintain equilibrium within this triangle. As an integral system, if one side gets sick, the other side will follow. To keep ourselves healthy is extremely important, because *health is freedom.*

Getting acquainted with medical history will better our understanding of disease. History is a great teacher, a reservoir of experience that unfolds the origin and vicissitudes of mankind.

It is hundreds of thousands of years ago and we are sleeping in a cave. Suddenly, a thunderclap wakes us up, lightning flashes, rain pours furiously, while hurricanes, tidal waves, and earthquakes modify the shape of continents. The sun rises and sets, the moon appears in different shapes, leaves fly away, snow falls, birds come back; then it is hot. The mysterious forces behind these events are unknown to us. Primitive humans witnessed hundreds of events that left them at the mercy of unknown forces. People had fever, pain, seizures, fractures, and became swollen or deranged. Leprosy broke the skin and deformed the face; cholera came with severe diarrhea and dehydration, killing people; malaria brought uncontrollable chills. Blindness, deafness, muteness, paralysis, a whole range of diseases overwhelmed us humans who were unable to explain why. We were defeated by superior forces.

We worshipped those forces and used magic, witchcraft, shamans, sorcerers, and religious sacrifices to keep the evil ones happy and away. Primitive people believed in visible and invisible natural phenomena as the cause of every wrongdoing, including disease. For them, diseases were caused by demons or worms, and death by evil eyes, gods, and stars. Witchcraft, religion, and medicine walked hand in hand for many centuries, alternating in popularity as treatments for the sick. Science was to replace the absolute of religion, magic, and quackery with the absolute of reasoning.

The Babylonians believed diseases were caused by gods. The priest physician was born, and magic, religion, and medicine were blended together in the search for answers to the causes of our illnesses. The Egyptians later developed two kinds of medicine; one rational and one magical. Finally, in the sixth century B.C., the Greeks began to understand why we got sick, and medicine flourished. The Middle Ages were a period of darkness in which no one explored the causes of illness, and once again disease was explained by the supernatural. Only within the last one hundred years have medical advancements taken place. We have moved away from myths, fantasy, and charlatanism into solid knowledge of how to treat diseases.

There is no single answer to why we become ill. Often it is because we break the laws of nature. If we don't take care of ourselves, we become weak and our defenses are reduced. At times, we are invaded and overpowered by the many bacteria that are on our skin and inside of us, on the walls of the digestive tract. If our defenses are intact, they cannot break through and make us ill.

Not long ago, surgeons when operating in the abdomen for various diseases often extirpated the appendix, even if it was normal. The belief was, let's prevent appendicitis and the need to have further surgery later on. Nowadays, the appendix is accepted as part of our lymphatic system's defense against disease. We must acknowledge that whatever is in our body has a reason to be there.

We have a unique capacity to get sick. Becoming ill jeopardizes our goals in life, our efforts to be integral beings. In this chapter we will review some of the causes of our illnesses, and those of the family, government, and society.

Tradition has divided diseases into two groups: mental and physical. The former was believed to be invisible, the latter, visible. In primitive times, because so little was known about the causes of illnesses, they were believed to be of divine or supernatural origin. Those who tried to inquire into other areas for causes of illnesses were jailed or even killed. The knowledge that diseases were caused by matter came as the result of the proposals of Democritus (460 to 350 B.C.), who stated that the universe, the body, and the soul were composed of invisible atoms. Based on this statement, Epicurus (341 to 270 B.C.) spoke of seeds that float in the air and produce diseases, but it took 1,800 years for Fracastoro of Verona to hint that infections were transmitted. A hundred years later, Van Leeuwenhoek (1632 to 1723) invented the microscope and began to examine the so-called invisible demons of the past. Two hundred years after that, Louis Pasteur revolutionized medicine by exposing the world of bacteria. During this same period, Lister's discovery of the properties of carbolic acid as an antiseptic allowed us to kill these microbes. This series of events closed a cycle in the historical evolution of knowledge about human disease.

Any organ may become diseased. Often a disease starts in one organ and spreads to others. Thus, the body mechanisms become affected, and our whole system is thrown out of balance. This loss of equilibrium may occur within minutes, as in serious bleeding, or it may take years to become noticeable, as in Parkinson's disease. During the course of an illness, our whole body is sick. An illness may last hours, days, or years. Time is an important factor: the longer an illness lasts, the more damage is done.

In 2,500 B.C. the Thracians advanced the concept that the body could not be healed without healing the soul. Nowadays psychosomatic medicine accepts that both the "emotional" and the "intellectual" brains may cause physical illnesses. Psychosomatic medicine has not recruited many followers among physicians, however, because they are not yet ready or willing to integrate body, emotions, and intellect under a single frame of reference. Nevertheless, we physicians recognize the psychosomatic components to diseases such as peptic ulcer, colitis, hypertension, asthma, heart ailments, obesity, acne, dermatitis, headaches, generalized pain, lower back pain, menstrual disorders, and hay fever. The list is extensive; it has been suggested, for example, that cancer may also have a psychosomatic component.

He was forty years old, happily married, two children, a successful executive, and he felt good about life. Then he began to complain of feeling sad, loss of appetite, fatigue, and insomnia. He consulted with a psychiatrist. A diagnosis of depression was made, and he was placed on antidepressants. Three months later, he felt worse and was admitted to a hospital for a complete checkup. An X ray of the abdomen revealed a mass that proved to be cancer of the pancreas. The man died. This was a case of an organic illness that manifested itself as a mental depression.

When an elderly person dies and the spouse dies soon afterward, we attribute the cause of death to heartache or loneliness. It has been proved that bereavement lowers the body's defenses. As a result of our emotions, we become more vulnerable to bodily disease or death.

We cannot divide the mind from the body when it comes to health. Whether it is a case of schizophrenia or bronchitis, we must examine both the body and the mind. If we consider this relationship, we will begin to see how perfectly assembled and organized we are, even in time of illness. We may be chopped up in the autopsy room, but never when we are alive. We only make sense as a whole. Therefore, when we look into our illness, we must look into its total impact on ourselves. The Romans said it first: "A sound mind in a sound body."

Our body utilizes a language common to every human—body language. To avoid misunderstandings, our body uses very reliable messengers—sounds, movements, pains, tears. Some never come out in the open and remain within our inner body. Others surface and can be observed by us. Physicians call these messengers symptoms, whose purpose it is to report the presence of illness. If we don't pay attention to our messages, they intensify until we do something about them. Because some of these messages may be more silent than others (for instance, the beginning of high blood pressure), we should go for a checkup once a year.

Our body was a Tower of Babel when we could not understand its messages. Sneezing, for example, meant that an evil spirit had left our body. Thereafter the practice of saying "God bless you," "Salud," and "Sihhaten" became a custom we still have, although we have forgotten the superstitious belief. Epileptic convulsions were another sign of demonic possession. In the Talmud, sweating, diarrhea, dreaming, and semen ejaculation were considered signs of a good recovery.

It is a good custom to be receptive to our own inner messengers. Every day we should look into our eyes, observe the color of our tongue, urine, and feces. The vital signs of pulse, blood pressure, and respiration are easy to check. These indicators may even tell you about the state of your emotions. For instance, hyperventilating or holding your breath is due to anxiety; increase of blood pressure is a consequence of anger; a speedy pulse or diarrhea is from fear or tension.

♦ ♦ ♦

Social Disease

A social disease is a disorder of the system that fails to provide the individual with the minimal necessities to preserve emotional and physical wellness. Societies become diseased when they fail to provide each individual with those things that are essential for health, such as food, proper housing, the availability of work, as well as time to play, and so forth.

For the average person, the recommended daily caloric intake is 2,500. However, millions of people live on starvation quotas of perhaps 160 calories per day. Famine has periodically devastated societies. In 1845 the Irish potato famine killed one million people, or 12.5 percent of the total population. Famine has taken countries to war. Moreover, it disrupts body growth, bringing up generations of deprived, underdeveloped children.

A room is an important part of our personal territory and freedom. Yet many are born and die with no roof over their heads. Others live jammed together in small quarters with a minimum of privacy. The result is illness.

Chagas' disease is an infection caused by *Trypanosoma cruzi*, a parasite living inside bloodsucking bugs that live in the thatched roofs of mud houses in rural areas of South America. At night they feed on the uncovered skin of sleeping people. It is estimated that over 25 percent of the population suffers from Chagas' disease, which causes a chronic inflammation of the heart. This condition may be dormant for many years but eventually causes disablement or death. This serious public health problem is an example of a diseased socioeconomic system directly affecting the individual.

Sanitary conditions are important to prevent infectious

diseases. Sir John Harrington, courtier and poet in the sixteenth-century court of Queen Elizabeth, invented the toilet (a distinct integration, poetry and sanitation!). Such an important artifact was not widely utilized until the end of the nineteenth century. Washing facilities, sewers, good light, and good ventilation in housing are essential to maintain health.

Industrialization of labor has brought extraordinary accomplishments, and along with these enough diseases to create a subspecialty of medicine: occupational health. Poisoning with heavy metals, such as lead, mercury, aluminum, arsenic, or toxic pesticides, is common. Lung diseases, such as black lung seen in miners, or radiation disease, for workers in nuclear facilities, indicate what is happening to us today.

One of the greatest threats to health in large cities is air contamination. Fuel is the main cause for air contamination, but now there is the additional threat to our health with the possibility of accidents in nuclear plants, such as those that occurred at Three Mile Island and Chernobyl.

Pleasure can also endanger our health. There are four major social diseases that result from our need to satisfy our appetite for pleasure: alcoholism, drug abuse, obesity, and venereal diseases.

Although alcohol can cause serious damage to our body, it is socially accepted throughout the world. Because alcohol has a long-standing tradition that goes back thousands of years, it is almost impossible to eradicate a habit so deeply rooted in every social class. The skyrocketing figures on alcoholism parallel the upward trend of economic depression, generalized poverty, suicide, and mental illness. Furthermore, there is tacit acceptance by governments to tolerate the promotion of alcohol consumption because alcohol taxation is an important source of revenue.

In modern warfare we do not need armed forces to conquer countries: we could destroy their inhabitants with amphetamines, angel dust, cocaine, marijuana, LSD, glue, gasoline, aspirins, morphine, sleeping pills, tranquilizers, and heroin. In fact, we could do what has been done to China and North Africa and many other regions of the world where people have been dominated by means of drugs. This is because drugs weaken our willpower, destroy our sense of duty, and chemically alter our metabolism.

What can society do about the drug problem? Very little. When the profit is so large and easily made, I don't foresee any immediate reason why those in charge of the drug market would quit. But we can do something about it as individuals and that is to refrain from using drugs by finding a meaning to life.

Obesity is rarely related to medical illnesses. Eating produces pleasure. Food is an accessible commodity that provides us with a cheap and fast return.

Many years ago I visited a bordello in the middle of nowhere in the Andean region. There, I met Madame Teodora, who had been a faithful worker for about thirty years. After inviting me for *pisco* (a strong alcoholic beverage of that region), she began to talk about her life. She was well known in the region, and very important people were regular clients of the bordello. She synthesized her success with a very short statement: "A good whore anticipates and influences the needs of her customers." It is no wonder that venereal diseases, too, are on the increase. When it comes to social diseases derived from pleasure, remedies are indeed difficult to find.

The increase in gambling, drug abuse, alcoholism, prostitution, venereal disease, depression, psychosomatic illness, violence, and social unrest, can be correlated to a decrease in moral and sexual values, productivity, interest in the arts, family unity, social solidarity, friendship, and individualism.

Do governments get sick? Governments get sick just as people, animals, and plants do.

If we add the number of the world rulers of 178 nations and multiply it by the average human body weight of 158 pounds, we have 28,124 pounds of flesh and bone. Thus it takes only 28,124 pounds of ruling flesh and bone to control 790,000 million pounds of citizens' flesh and bones.

A government is like a human body, made up of cells; each cell is an officer of the government. A government is a live body subjected to diseases like the rest of us, the diseases of poverty, inflation, or totalitarianism. In each case the government has lost its equilibrium. Governments talk about a "healthy" market, a "depressed" economy, the "ills" of our time, a "moral" commitment, and so on. Perhaps unconsciously the government has accepted being a gigantic human body. A diseased government will affect the society it rules. All the inhabitants will suffer from the illness. For instance, inflation spreads like the flu, becomes an epidemic, and depletes your resources and defenses.

Here are some symptoms of a diseased government:

1. Failure to have free elections.
2. Failure to allow blank ballots to be used by voters who dislike candidates.
3. Presence of war, revolution, guerrillas.

4. Presence of political prisoners, killings, torture, missing people.
5. Presence of strikes due to unfair labor practices.
6. Lack of policy based on humanistic principles of mutual respect and individual freedom.
7. Monopoly of the mass media.
8. Censorship.
9. Withholding information from the people.
10. Unfair distribution of taxes.
11. Inflation.
12. A decrease of funds for health, education, and peaceful research.
13. Influence by the military on political processes.
14. Presence of embezzlement.
15. Moral corruption.

Keep in mind the concept of a diseased government because it may help to explain why life is hard for the average person in that country. The average person has little to say in the public life of a country, so if the country holds elections, it will provide a chance for the individual to speak up. The active participation of all in public affairs should be a matter of duty. Maybe then we will reverse wrongdoing and cure the disease of the government. We all know it is very convenient to sit back, relax, and watch our favorite TV programs, but we shouldn't pass our lives this way. Our life script belongs only to us, and we must be writer, director, and actor in it.

··· Chapter Ten

THE ART OF HEALING

> If all drugs were dumped into the sea, it would be the best thing ever to happen to mankind and the worst to happen to fishes.
>
> Oliver Wendell Holmes, quoted in B. L. Gordon, *The Romance of Medicine* (1949)

As soon as we become ill we are hit by uncertainty: what is wrong with me? If we don't know, fear sets in; if our malady is untreatable, we despair. To avoid these feelings, we have learned how to heal.

Because the universe and individuals are made of earth, air, water, and fire, the healer has always looked to these four elements to treat disease. Primitive people learned from the healing instincts of animals, which use grass, mud, and saliva as remedies. The basic medicines were air, water, stone, salt, mud, and fire.

The ancients believed in the breath of life, that the air from the lungs had curative properties. In the Middle East, a mother will gently breathe on her child's wound. In modern medicine, the use of oxygen in therapy is well accepted. In the Hebrides Islands, salt was eaten to produce dreams revealing the future. Fire, in the form of a branding iron, was used to stop bleeding; as a heat cup, it was used to decongest the lungs. The electrical surgical knife is a modern version of the use of fire in medicine.

As animals will cover a broken limb with mud, so once did we. Mud from certain regions is still used for general healing purposes, mainly for the treatment of diseases of the skin and joints. At the Ganges River and in the grotto of Lourdes miraculous cures are still attributed to water. Medicinal water, due to its chemical properties, is still popular around the world.

It was once a custom to place a child suffering from rickets in the forked branch of an ash tree facing the sun, although no one knew that rickets, a deficiency of vitamin D, required exposure to sunlight as a corrective. Iron was given for anemia as early as 700 B.C. In the sixteenth century, Paracelsus used magnets to drain unwanted accumulations of fluids from organs. Research in the use of magnetic fields to treat illness goes on today.

An early belief was that the body could be cured by applying substances possessing shapes or colors similar to the afflicted part or illness. The rash of measles could be relieved by covering the skin with a red blanket. It was acceptable to rub one's gums with the finger of a dead person to kill a toothache. To prevent colds or leg cramps, knots were make in clothes and handkerchiefs.

Blood, the most vital element, also played a role. It was drunk in potions, injected under the skin, and even removed from the body. The Incas had already transfused blood by the time Giovanni Colle of Italy put transfusion into practice in 1628. Until this century, bloodletting was a common form of treatment. Barber-surgeons would hang a sheet stained with blood at their shop doors to indicate the opening of the bloodletting season.

The Egyptians were the first to challenge legend and superstition in medicine and bring a more rational approach to it. They used vapors to treat uterine bleeding by placing the patient, legs spread, above boiling urine. The Egyptians believed that urine vapors would stop the bleeding. Today we know that urea, a substance present in urine, has clotting properties.

Hippocrates (460 to 377 B.C.), a Greek physician considered the father of medicine, also did not believe in legends. He said that we are each a composite of earth, air, fire, and water, and that health depends upon an adequate proportion of these elements. Hippocrates' contributions to medicine include studies in anatomy, disease, diagnosis, prognosis, and treatment by drugs and diets. He formulated the rules of medical ethics, which led to the Hippocratic Oath. In addition, Hippocrates pioneered the hypothesis that the human temperament is regulated by body fluids. Today it is accepted that body chemistry is related to the mechanisms of some mental disorders.

Historically, the brain has been a no-man's-land. As a consequence, it has been subjected to many kinds of atrocities perpetrated under the noble guise of "cure." We have listened, spoken to, suggested, commanded, and hypnotized the brain. The brain has been chained in asylums, burned by witch hunters, chopped by surgeons, and electroshocked by psychiatrists. The brain remains one of the least understood organs.

Attempts to treat the brain as an integral part of the body were carried out in the Greek town of Epidaurus in the fourth century B.C. A shrine for Asclepius, the god of healing, was erected there in the shape of a maze where depressed patients were bathed, massaged, given food, wine, and music. During sleep, a god would appear in their dreams and a cure was obtained. Although the Greeks knew that wine made them happy, they didn't know that it contains phenylethylamine, a mood regulator, which might have helped.

Dreaming was also used to heal. Many centuries ago, we did not know what to make of dreams, and we were fascinated and scared of this inner world. The Egyptians were the first to interpret the meaning of dreams.

For hundreds of years, psychiatry remained in the hands of priests, pagans, quacks, and witches. It was in the seventeenth and eighteenth centuries that demonology moved out and medicine moved in, once again, to treat the mentally ill. The power of suggestion was put forth by Mesmer and the concept of the unconscious mind by Fechner. Sexual repression, a subject unacceptable to neurologists, was later masterfully unfolded by Freud.

If the origin of illness was believed to be found in gods, planets, and demons, the treatment was directed toward those causes. The logic was to appease or chase out those powerful forces that made our lives miserable. For that reason, we worshipped, prayed, sang, danced, and offered human and animal sacrifices to those who seemed to be the cause of disease. We also fasted and whipped ourselves night and day with the single objective of being healthy. Shamans, sorcerers, exorcists, medicine men, witches, priests, and psychics shared the responsibility for curing us.

On the other hand, at different periods in time the origin of illness was ascribed to rational causes devoid of legend and superstition. This stand resulted in the presence of new members in the trade of healing, among them barbers, surgeons, physicians, naturopaths, osteopaths, chiropractors, homeopaths, psychiatrists, psychologists, pharmacists, and sociologists, all of whom claimed to know the answers. Thus, a diseased individual has, in fact, two dangers to face:

one, the illness; the other, the healer. Whether we like it or not, there is a type of disease called iatrogenic, which is caused by the healer, or by the medicine itself.

In 1982, one million people worldwide died as a result of medication side effects. The same year the international pharmaceutical industry reported 90 billion dollars in sales. We should recognize that, when ill, we are in jeopardy of losing our freedom as we surrender ourselves to healers. Many practitioners still walk the twilight path of incomplete knowledge; therefore, for our own sake, let us not forget how the practice of healing has evolved throughout history.

Healing is an art: it requires creativity, observation, study, and experience. Four requirements are needed to heal: identification of the illness, choice of the right treatment, prognosis, and compassion.

The best healers are those who combine scientific and empirical wisdom with love toward the patient. The old prescription of tenderness, love, and care is still valid. It strengthens the doctor-patient relationship, and it facilitates recovery.

A good healer treats the individual rather than the disease. Because it is the individual who has lost his or her balance; the disease is a consequence.

An illness impacts on our self-pride. We feel embarrassed; we see illness as a sign of weakness. We feel impotent, due to our inability to cope with it, or our failure to avoid it.

An integral being accepts illness as part of being a conscious living organism. An illness is not punishment. We must face illness with courage.

The integral being knows that healing is a self-directed phenomenon: we heal ourselves with our own inner resources. The outside healer or physician is merely an assistant. For instance, the cast on our broken leg keeps the bone in place while the bone heals itself. We must have a confident, committed attitude toward our illness. Otherwise, the healing process might remain unfinished.

A few questions should be asked before we embark on the journey to healing.

What illness do I have?

I am told I have a peptic ulcer, but I also know that everything started by keeping my anger inside. Should I treat my anger as well?

Why did I become ill?

It is of utmost relevance to trace the illness's origins and precipitating factors. An illness is a warning calling for a reexamination of life-style.

How did I become ill?

To know the ways an illness operates will bring understanding and acceptance of the illness and will help outline a healing strategy.

Am *I* an illness?

Some individuals prefer to be the illness rather than to have one. This affects their attitude toward the illness. How can we get rid of an illness if we are the illness? We are not illnesses.

How do I go about healing?

Because healing requires tremendous binding of the body and mind, we have to open all our avenues of energy, thoughts, and feelings, so the flow of our self will not remain obstructed by the disease. We call upon our self-reliance and our determination to restore our health.

What is the best healing system?

An integral being is insightful and open-minded and searches for the best therapy to be cured. Orthodox therapies are conservative and cautious; new ideas are accepted only when they have been scientifically proved. Sometimes this attitude may impede the introduction of new healing concepts as the orthodox healer continues to heal with obsolete methods.

The integral being should not feel limited to orthodox medical options to heal what has been damaged. We have the duty to explore, inquire, compare, and decide about what seems to be the most reasonable treatment approach.

Alternative therapies are options to be considered. From Chinese medicine to manipulative or paranormal therapies, a whole range is available. In many circumstances orthodox and alternative therapies can complement each other. The idea is not to praise one system of healing and condemn the other. The idea is to integrate the best of each and put them to work together to treat the integral being.

We should not make the mistake of believing that primitive people only used magic, legend, and pure nonsense to treat illnesses. Not at all! Our ancestors had creativity and imagination that have not yet been surpassed in modern times. Regrettably, we show contempt for a past that we have misunderstood and misjudged. It would be to our advantage to look back into the ancient traditions of medicine to extract wisdom we might apply today.

In spite of fate, omens, augurs, quackery, and medications that may kill instead of cure, we have made tremendous progress in the art of healing. Nevertheless, new diseases are just around the corner: viruses become fat on antibiotics, epidemics continue to sweep countries, famine kills as usual, and we are as violent as ever. What has happened? We have not been treated in an integral manner, taking into consideration our body, intellect, and emotions.

Does everyone accept healing easily?

The most difficult area I have encountered in my practice as a physician is the resistance of the patient to treatment. Leaving aside emergencies, such as serious injuries, heart attacks, and seizures, the natural tendency of a patient is to postpone the visit to the doctor. Before seeing a doctor, the patient will try the advice of family and friends, over-the-counter drugs, folklore medicine, praying, or resort to a wait-and-see attitude. Worsening of symptoms, bleeding, or uncontrollable pain are factors that force the patient to make a trip to a doctor's office. Among the mentally ill, the refusal to see a psychiatrist may prolong the duration of treatment or make the illness chronic.

The denial of an illness is the result of self-destructive behavior. The presence of a disease brings upon us a fear of impending death. It awakens the dormant feeling that we can die anytime. A disease imposes an unpleasant reality that forces us to center within ourselves. Most of us abhor unpleasantness and cannot bear to be centered in our own life.

Our tendency to procrastinate with our health is disheartening. Procrastination is epitomized by the woman who discovers a lump in her breast and decides against a medical consultation. She chooses to live in the hope that it is benign and that it will magically vanish. Procrastination is the obese man who suffers from diabetes and high blood pressure and has been told that his main arteries will burst and he will have a brain hemorrhage if he keeps eating the way he does. His response is to keep indulging himself with cake and ice cream.

Although most people start some sort of treatment, few people remain in it. About half of all medical prescriptions never arrive at the drugstore. It could be argued that many symptoms vanish by the time we get to the pharmacy. We could also say that some symptoms are psychological and disappear without treatment. Unfortunately, these are not really the reasons; instead, it is because we tend to procrastinate. A pill or a visit to the doctor is a reminder that we have an illness.

Of all the chapters I have written, this one suits me best. I am a healer, I was born a healer, and I expect to die one, only giving up to face my death. I was six years old when I found a picture of a bearded female in a medical book. That was, I believe, the beginning of my vocation. Then, the death of my mother and a series of childhood diseases drew me closer to the field of medicine. I could never see the anguish of my patients without being moved. I never saw eyes more inquisitive than those of severely ill patients looking into mine in search of a hopeful sign. Their hopes became mine. Today I look back and see old hospital corridors, beds lined up in endless wards, the smell of antiseptic, infections, and death. I remember anatomy amphitheaters, silent morgues, the chronic lament of the emergency room, the gushing of blood in the operating room, the last rite of closing eyelids. It is a frightening and overwhelming responsibility to take care of a human life.

As a healer, I have always refused to become a witness to my patient's suffering; I have always chosen to be a participant. The healer who becomes so involved in the process of healing eventually wears out. Yet how could I remain detached from my patient's pain?

Early on, I was exposed to the arts of preventive medicine and healing within my own family environment. I had the opportunity to see and try what were then considered traditional methods of therapy as well as unconventional approaches. Herbal teas and vitamins for colds, mud therapy for skin rejuvenation, tonics for the brain, oils for hair growth, walking barefoot in a puddle of cold water to liberate energy, eating honeycomb to remain young, drinking red meat juice to grow strong, and taking cod liver oil to prevent weakness were all part of the array of choices available to improve one's health.

As my godfather was teaching internal medicine at the university hospital, my aunt would recommend the application of sliced cold potatoes on our temples to relieve a headache if aspirins failed to do the job. There was plenty of knowledge in our household, and perhaps because of that there was the flexibility to try new modes of making our lives more meaningful and healthy.

In 1968, the winner of two Nobel prizes, Linus Pauling, wrote an article in *Science* stating that mental diseases should be treated by providing the optimum molecular environment for the mind, especially the optimum concentration of substances normally present in the human body. Here was someone speaking of equilibrium between the molecules, the mind, the body. The concept made sense and echoed my own ideas about mental illness or any other illness, namely, the loss of equilibrium.

After twenty years I became frustrated with my profession. I could not tolerate just being a pill-pusher and a sympathetic ear. I wanted action. I wanted to be a better healer. I went back to my medicine books and looked for links between the body and the mind. A new panorama opened as I began to integrate my approach to medicine. I would not only listen to my patients' problems, but I would also give them a physical examination.

Advancements in the field of biological psychiatry were taking place, and I was pleased to participate in these avenues of research. I began to experiment with diets, vitamins, minerals, and amino acids. Some of our nutritional research was satisfactory, but by 1972 I was no longer satisfied. Patients who had improved wanted more. What could I do? I was at a turning point in my career. I began to talk more to my patients—but this time I talked about their attitudes, behavior, and life-styles.

If a patient needs talk therapy I prefer to apply common sense to resolve the immediate needs. Long-term therapy, such as psychoanalysis, does not offer prompt solutions. Moreover, while resolving current problems new ones appear and the backlog becomes unbearable. The ideal program of talk therapy should be focused on the here and now. My question was which psychological treatment would fit my patients' needs best? Thinking about these issues I decided to incorporate behavioral therapy in an effort toward an integral approach to psychiatry. The idea was to help people to become more assertive and productive. In the meantime we could work at a slower-paced program to apply common sense and knowledge and to develop awareness.

Throughout the years I have stayed aware of the need to improve health care and forms of treatments. While working in Buenos Aires, I noticed that some of my patients were outspoken about social issues such as inflation, the uncertainty of the future, and the power struggle going on among the ruling classes of Argentina. I observed that these patients were more difficult to treat. Other patients, facing political persecution, manifested higher degrees of anxiety or depression. In such instances, I provided them with medication and a sympathetic ear. But was that enough?

I knew that the social environment affects our internal chemistry and body functions. So the question was: If the cause was social, what good did it do to minister to the brain to keep the internal environment in equilibrium? Wouldn't it be better to start with the external environment—providing social justice—and then readjust the brain and its internal environment?

I began to discuss this concept with my patients. Associating their illness with social factors became a fundamental element in their recovery. I began to sense that social psychiatry had a major place in mental health programs. The challenge was how to implement it in treatment programs.

Another influential period of my development as a healer took place while working in Bedford-Stuyvesant, a ghetto neighborhood in Brooklyn, New York. There I came into direct contact with victims of hunger, drugs, and a minority subculture that shook many of my conceptions about the fairness of the American distribution of wealth, education, and health.

The problems of the Bedford-Stuyvesant patients were just about impossible to handle. What was the priority? The fever, the hunger, the fix, the despair, the loneliness, the rage, or the fear? Under those bleak circumstances, my prescription pad became useless. What kind of a healer was I supposed to be? I felt impotent, unable to help, and embarrassed because I had more than they had. But I am grateful to those patients because they made me aware of what social medicine was all about.

I thought it would be important to work with a team—psychiatrists, psychologists, nurses, social workers, art therapists, and research assistants. This group of professionals would share a common goal: to better themselves as therapists by offering a more comprehensive therapeutic program. This program included a physical examination, laboratory tests, psychological evaluation, and a psychosocial history.

I had one patient who was ready for our rehabilitation program. Therefore, I requested a session with his family. During it, I noticed that his mother was rather reluctant to accept the idea that her son was to be discharged. "I am afraid he'll relapse," she said. Nonetheless, he was discharged, but one month later he was back for treatment. What had happened?

The patient explained that his mother did not allow him to participate in the rehabilitation program out of fear that the "sick people in the program would not be a good example" for her son. While I had been ready to discharge him, the patient's mother was not ready. She had dedicated her life to the care of a son who was schizophrenic. What was she going to do with her own life if I cured him?

The importance of family therapy was proven. But now I had further questions. How important was the economic background of the patient?

When patients skip their medication because they cannot afford to buy it, when patients do not follow a wholesome diet because starches and sweets are cheaper, I see the importance of having jobs, money, a good welfare system, and a society that cares. It is pathetic when a patient cannot afford consultation. Poor people neglect their health.

I learned that healing requires integration of the internal and external environment. It is the healer's job to take all of those factors into consideration in order to recover health or prevent disease.

··· Chapter Eleven

THE ART OF PREVENTION

> . . . and do you want me to come back to check my blood pressure? What's the matter with you?!
>
> A patient

We all face the daily ongoing struggle to maintain health and fight off disease. We have learned through trial and error how to do this. In the past, water glasses had lids to keep demons out; there were forbidden rivers, lakes, and ponds that were said to be inhabited by demons. Probably these waters were sources of dysentery and typhoid fever.

Jews and Moslems were forbidden to eat pork on religious grounds. Pork can carry the cyst of a parasite difficult to kill even with today's technology. The shamans of Turkey would fumigate the clothes and merchandise of travelers from abroad to neutralize evil forces. They were practicing what is known today as quarantine.

In order to keep ourselves healthy we seek to control the forces of expansion (growth), of reduction (aging), and of aggression (life). A healthy life requires a program easy to remember and to follow. We need a good diet, physical exercise, rest, and intellectual and emotional balance.

We have to set short-term and long-term goals. At the start of our program we may adopt a "just for today" attitude. Gradually we'll realize that we can become accustomed to this new life-style, and if we skip some of our program's activities we will miss them. In addition, if we begin to follow an irregular schedule, our body will respond with "withdrawal symptoms," such as fatigue, weight gain, irritability, and disturbed sleep. The lesson here is that we can become addicted to a healthy life-style and that a return to old habits will not be silently accepted by our body.

There are four contributory factors that determine our life span: hereditary traits, nutrition, stress prevention, and medical care. These factors are our partners in the business of keeping healthy. With the exception of hereditary, we can modify the other factors as we please. To live longer, we must take sole responsibility.

Our program should have imagination, creativity, motivation, and stimulation. As individuals, let's put a touch of our own inventiveness to work.

Daily Menu for the Body

Let us design a strategy of prevention, a few daily measures to keep our organism fit. One way of doing it is to verify that our body's messengers are sending healthy signals. To do this, we must get acquainted with our patterns of behavior: posture, movement, and physiological activities (eating, sleeping, and so on). Assuming we have normal patterns of body behavior, any deviation from the norm may require further investigation.

The best way to examine your body is to stand naked in front of a mirror. Is your posture correct, or do you slouch? Does your head sink between your shoulders? Do you have a potbelly or bulges? Are you able to hold your body in an erect position, even when you are seated? A bad posture keeps your frame misaligned, straining your muscles and subsequently modifying the tension of tissues and the position of the organs inside your body. Many physical ailments are directly related to posture or bone disorders. Do you ever wonder why the armed forces emphasize good posture? A good posture reflects your stance in life, your self-reliance, determination, willpower, and readiness to face the struggle for life.

The way we walk and sit, our gestures, the position we assume to sleep—in general, our motions—are the mechanical expressions of our character.

When you awaken ask yourself whether you have had a good or bad night's sleep. Restless? Bad dreams or nightmares? Check your muscles: are they tight or relaxed? Do you already feel tired? Do you dread getting up and starting a new day, or are you ready to spring out of bed and conquer the world?

Some people need extra time to wake up. They get up, but they act like zombies. Not all of us operate on the same daily clock. Some are night people, who perform best in the evenings; others are day people, who perform their best in the morning. People should contemplate the possibility of accommodating their work schedules to their biological clock. Some companies allow workers to choose their own shifts to improve performance.

When you wake up, your body is ready to begin its daily dialogue with you. Don't ignore it, converse—you are partners in life. In the bathroom, look at yourself in the mirror. Check your eyelids: are they swollen? Are your eyes red? Do you have circles around your eyes? How is your skin? Pale? Reddish? Bluish? Normal? Stick out your tongue. Is it of a normal pink, or is it coated white? Check your gums.

Pale, soft? Bleeding gums are indicators of several problems (poor dental care, poor nutrition, stress). By the way, do you grind or clench your teeth during sleep? If yes, ask yourself how tense you are before falling asleep. An easy way to check is by opening your mouth wide and seeing if your jaws hurt. Tension can remain during sleep if you don't go to bed fully relaxed.

Everyone should periodically check their feces and urine, since changes in these waste products may indicate internal disturbances. A black or red color in feces may hint at the possibility of intestinal or rectal bleeding. One drop of blood can tint your urine red. Tea-colored urine may indicate liver troubles. If you see any changes in the external appearance of your body or in your urination, defecation, or menstruation habits, you should consult a physician.

Now that you are groomed and dressed, you are ready for breakfast. Perhaps you are not hungry in the morning, or you are trying to lose weight, or you have no time for breakfast. If your last meal was the evening before, those twelve hours or more without food will have caused a decrease in your blood sugar. Therefore, as soon as you are on the go, you will begin to feel tired, irritable, anxious, or all of these. The best time to assimilate food is in the morning, so a good breakfast is a must. Try to avoid the typical coffee and doughnut start. Sweets and more than one cup of coffee elevate your blood sugar level, but in three hours you will experience a precipitous drop in sugar and feel tired. A good breakfast may include fruit juice, yogurt, whole cereals, milk, toast, and cheese.

Now you are ready to face the world. How well you are able to do this will be determined by your attitude and response to your external environment. It pays to look at the sky, whether you live in the city, the suburbs, or on a farm. We look at the sky to remind ourselves that we too are part of the universe. A blue sky and a sunny day are symbols of the nutrition that descends to earth from the sun and the air. A cloudy sky means that water is coming to feed our land and our vegetation. The sky is never "gloomy," if we view it properly.

Even if we have been following the same route to work for years, we should observe our surroundings. Observing our environment sharpens our brain. When we are out in the street, we must actively participate in our environment. The street is the most important showcase of social life, habits, and behaviors of a people. Everything is to be seen there—the way people move, shapes, color, cars, the windows of the stores, the street vendors, and so forth. It all provides an impression of the totality of life.

The diseases of society also show up in the street. Dirty streets with uncollected waste are indicators of deeper problems. If we fear walking at night, if we have given muggers and rapists ownership of the streets, we know we have a diseased society. On our way to work, can we cope with all this? Can we take the noise, the pandemonium, the chaos of rush hour? Sometimes we can't; we are too tired, too worried. "It has gotten to me" we say. However, on other days, the infernal noise sounds like music, the pandemonium is exciting, and the rush-hour chaos a challenge. We are happy, we feel good, we can tolerate things as they are. We know this by paying attention to our body cues, because they monitor how we are doing when we walk or ride about our town.

Some pedestrians resort to Walkmans and some drivers will shut out sound in their cars to avoid social contact. It is not good to dull your senses to outside noise; it will take you nowhere. If anything, you will end up becoming an isolated being.

Courtesy can make everyday life easier for all of us. Why mention it, if everyone knows it? Well, we may know it, but we may not practice it. Being courteous is the best way to interact with others because courtesy indicates respect for others. We have learned that mutual respect is essential for us to live together in freedom. What better way to show our acceptance of freedom than by being polite to one another? Our world belongs to us, and we must be responsible for it.

As we enter our homes, it is best not to carry in our work problems. It will be difficult to relax and communicate with others. If you feel tense about work, try to get some time for yourself. We need to talk to ourselves, analyze who we are and what we want.

At the end of the day, relax, exercise, or go for a walk. Drinking dulls your intellect and only postpones your worries. Martini people should have only one. Moderation is extremely important in the integration process.

Food for Your Body

A century and a half after Brillat-Savarin said, "Show me what you eat and I will tell you who you are," we are beginning to accept the indivisible bond established between food and our chemical makeup. Yet, how few of us are truly aware of this! Nowadays, we eat what becomes available—food impregnated with chemicals ranging from color dyes to insecticides and radiation. The prospect of having to go through life accepting poison as food is madness.

For the integral being, bread is the symbol by which we marry nature. Bread requires the four basic elements: soil for the grain, water for the flour, air for the yeast, and fire for the cooking. To eat bread is an important ceremony and as such should be performed seriously.

If we want to live in health, we need a revision of our eating habits. If we have doubts about it, let's remember the English proverb that says, "The glutton digs his grave with his teeth."

Nutritional requirements vary with age and special needs such as pregnancy, lactation, or those of specific diseases. When we are babies, we should each begin our education in the advantages of good nutrition. Our parents should train us to develop an acceptable pattern of eating behavior. We must learn how to eat the right foodstuffs and how to avoid under- or overeating. The nutritional needs of children are determined by their growth and development.

With age, we sustain hormonal and metabolic changes and have different nutritional needs. In general, there is a slowdown of our physical functions. The older person will benefit by taking lighter and smaller but more frequent meals, since there is also a slowdown of the digestive process.

For vegetarians, knowledge about protein sources is a must, because the main protein source, found in meat, is not acceptable. Additional precautions should be exerted by vegetarians who use laxatives or enemas, who practice fasting, or who restrict intake of fluids. Attention to nutritional needs should be especially heeded by vegetarian pregnant women and children under the age of two. Vegetarians have to obtain good sources of high-quality proteins, calcium, iron, and vitamins B-2 and B-12.

An eating plan should consider our personal eating habits and preferences but should also consider budget limitations. In order to maintain a healthy diet, we must understand the food-body relationship. This will be the best step toward proper nutrition. Books on diets and health and budget and diets are available in public libraries and bookstores. To become educated in these matters is a plus for our health.

Guidelines for a Good Diet

1. Plenty of vegetables, salads, white meats over red meats, dairy products (yogurt over milk), and whole cereals.
2. Avoid salt, sugar products, and processed carbohydrates.
3. Raw vegetables and fresh fruits are excellent for their vitamin content, easy digestion, and as aids against constipation.
4. Chew food slowly.
5. To avoid excessive dilution of the digestive juices, drink fewer liquids with meals.

For the Overweight

1. Use willpower.
2. Use physical exercise.
3. Use smaller plates.
4. Leave utensils on the plate between mouthfuls.
5. Remember that it takes twenty minutes to feel full after eating, so eat slowly.
6. Do not snack.
7. Keep calm.
8. Reward yourself with anything but food.
9. Eat only at your dinner table, not at different locations around the house.

Care of the Intellect

In the same manner that we feed our body, we have to feed our intellect. The intellect develops and grows like any other organ of the body. A harmonious intellect will be our courier to the world. Do not lock your future in a narrow mind. Let it grow, and take care of it. Just as you develop a program for the care of your body there is a daily care program for your brain. The technique is threefold: reading, thinking, and memory exercises.

By reading, we prevent ignorance from becoming a negative force in our development. To be mindful of events taking place requires the acquisition of information. Reading keeps us away from intellectual stagnation. A rusty brain does not belong to an integral being. A good book, like a good companion, brings happiness to our moments of loneliness.

Reading is the most important tool for developing our intellectual capacities. We exercise our learning capacity, our ability to associate, differentiate, and compare. Reading stimulates abstract and concrete thinking. Reading forces us to judge and give opinions, boosting our imagination, ideas, and dreams. Reading opens doors to the world of knowledge, and, as we already know, without knowledge freedom becomes an unreachable goal. Gathering information puts our intelligence to work. Give yourself a chance: READ!

To prevent is, in a way, to preserve. Integral beings preserve their thinking. Good thinking is a hallmark of a well-balanced individual.

Productive thinking is inquisitive and independent, challenging and in-depth. However, our everyday thinking is rapid and superficial, which is partly a consequence of our long-term training. We are accustomed to conforming and obeying without too much questioning. Furthermore, the mass media constantly makes up our minds for us. Therefore, we operate and respond in an environment of impoverished thought and automatic behavior. Yet who wants predigested thoughts?

We preserve our thinking by taking care of our brain and maintaining a balanced body-mind interplay.

One of our goals in life is to do a reasonable amount of independent thinking. Independent thinkers take nothing for granted, and preserve their freedom of mind. To think is a personal and private task. We may be physically jailed, but our thoughts will remain at liberty.

The mere thought that our memory is going to fail is anxiety provoking. To begin to forget names, dates, events, and so forth can be frightening. Memory loss is generally seen in organic disorders of the brain and in aging. Otherwise, memory impairment is uncommon. What is common is our inability to pay attention when we are under severe stress. A shorter attention span prevents us from registering and storing ongoing events. When we try to retrieve those events from our memory storage nothing shows up because nothing has been stored.

Some people may experience memory difficulties because they are no longer utilizing certain memory functions. For instance, electronic calculators are replacing our capacity to perform mathematical tasks.

Tips for Improving Memory

1. Pay attention. Avoid distraction.
2. An exercise: Make a mental note of all the objects present in a room. Leave the room and write down the

name of all the objects. Come back and see how much you remember.
3. Memorize poetry.
4. Avoid the use of calculators for simple mathematical tasks.
5. Do not attempt to learn when anxious; you will not retain information that never registered.

Care of the Emotions

Emotions are stimulated by positive and negative information arriving at our brains. We may preserve our emotional balance by screening out negative elements. To control our emotions, we must know ourselves well. Sometimes negative emotions settle in such a subtle way that they go undetected, as chronic knots do in our muscles. Furthermore, some individuals choose suffering as a way of life, refusing to change or procrastinating change. When this occurs, it is difficult to evaluate ourselves. We must do a lot of introspection and observe our behavior.

Somewhere between the intellect and the emotions is the spiritual zone. No matter what we believe, this spiritual region needs as good care as the rest of us. For some, the spiritual region is composed of high moral values without religious connotation. For others, walking into a house of worship brings an immediate feeling of serenity and security.

It is a lack of spiritual values that permits the present world situation to worsen. Sometimes we are embarrassed to admit the need for spirituality. However, we are all struggling on the same earth. Anything that may be beneficial to us should be utilized, as long as we don't hurt others or ourselves. Nonetheless, you should not expect

God to do your work for you. As the samurai said, "Believe in the gods, but do not depend upon them."

Menu for the Emotions

1. Meditate half an hour every day.
2. Read one poem daily.
3. Write down your emotions, perhaps your own poetry.
4. Draw or paint.
5. Learn a craft.
6. Read works on spiritual subjects.
7. Take walks.
8. Explore forests, look at landscapes, walk by rivers and oceans.
9. Learn how to laugh.
10. Sing, whistle, dance.
11. Watch a funny show or read the comics every day.
12. Develop honest and satisfying relations with relatives and friends.

Theoretically, the modern human being should be able to live 125 years. We are far from that goal, and stress appears to be the major obstacle to living longer. Stress is like an aggressor that invades our boundaries, whether mental or physical. These invaders, as in any war, have specific targets in our body, usually our "weak parts."

I basically classify stressors according to their position within our life span. Areas of stress include disappointment, work pressure, lack of time, substance abuse, disease, and major social, family, and emotional events, such as weddings, divorces, death, war. Within a social context, the main cause of stress in modern society is the human being, the major architect of stressors.

Stress causes a variety of symptoms: eyelid twitches, headache, teeth grinding, jaw clenching, neck pain, lower back pain, muscle twitches, tremors, cough, chest pains, fatigue, tension, irritability, insomnia, inability to make decisions, inability to complete a thought, loss of memory, loss of libido, loss of interest, anger, intolerance, anxiety, depression, and mood swings. Some diseases, such as high blood pressure, myocardial infarction, peptic ulcer, colitis, cancer, and premature aging, have been known to be stress-related diseases.

An excellent way of controlling our mental and physical balance and reducing stress is by practicing meditation. Meditation is a mental exercise that allows us to look slowly and calmly inwardly on important subjects of our lives. Meditation, together with praying, has been an important component of religious and mystical experience; consequently, many schools of meditation have developed.

The aim of religious or mystical meditation is to transcend beyond the material into the spiritual world. One arrives at that stage by gaining knowledge and understanding about oneself and one's surroundings. Regardless of religious aims, we can all use meditation to improve our present human condition, based on our reality and our acceptance of being part of the universe. Meditation can be a powerful tool to help us think without rushing, by forcing us to break our daily routines. Furthermore, meditation can be helpful to improve or maintain our body's physiology. It has been reported that it relieves high blood pressure and migraines, lowers cholesterol, slows down the heartbeat, improves sleep disorders, and reduces tension and stress.

If possible, meditation should be practiced twice daily, preferably at the beginning and end of the day for about twenty to thirty minutes each time. To meditate we should choose a quiet room and make arrangements to avoid being disturbed. Although most people utilize the traditional lotus position to meditate, any other position that makes us comfortable should suffice. Subdued lighting will enhance the silence; a candle will help us focus our minds on one single object or subject. Music also helps us to meditate.

For a meditation exercise, let us walk into the universe. We look at the candle and its beams. We absorb the candle's light through our semiclosed eyes, creating a new symphony of light and shape. If we have a piece of crystal we can look at the candle flame through it, designing new images of lights and shadows. We allow ourselves to diffuse our mind inside the light, and the flow of our thoughts becomes the flow of the flame. Remember, we are also fire.

In a second meditation exercise, we lie down and listen to music. We empty ourselves of every possible thought. Then we walk into the music; we let the music invade our brain. We substitute a thought with a melody. We become any of the instruments being played. The sounds of music travel in space, where they bounce against planets and interact with other lights and sounds. We are in space, visiting other territories, getting away from boundaries, clocks, and fears. We begin to sense a feeling of security and peace. An absolute peace pervades our senses and our flesh. We realize we need nothing. Past and future are gone. We live for the instant, the magic instant of our fusion with the universe. It is then when we realize how futile are lives lived devoid of universal experience.

In a third exercise, we switch off the music and put out the candle. We are ready to meditate about specific subjects. Many times problems can be resolved by meditation. What meditation brings to us is a general feeling of well-being, a sense of inner peace, and an improved ability to interact with people, control stress, and look at a suffering world with understanding and love.

Meditation is a difficult exercise to carry out. When we wake up in the morning we rush out of the house to attend to our obligations. When we return from work we just want to go to sleep and forget. How can we be in the mood to explore inner peace after a day of conforming to the rules of the game of surviving?

"I have no time to sit and relax and meditate." A response I have heard thousands of times. We keep denying the reality of our existence. If we do not have time for ourselves, who will? We are sacred, and whether we like it or not sacred objects are to be worshipped and cared for. We are walking temples in which the universe dwells. Yes, right inside us.

A good fitness program has to be complete, reasonable, practical, and easy to implement. A successful program is based on discipline, perseverance, and patience. We should be able to perform the program without the use of equipment; thus, we will not have excuses when we are away on business trips or on vacation.

Exercise has a positive effect on the body-mind connection, stress, weight control, body image, and self-confidence. It increases the calcium content of our bones, builds up a better heart pump, and increases the good HDL cholesterol. Physical fitness also prevents muscle loss, and keeps joints mobile and supple.

The interaction between muscles and emotion is another important aspect of your body. You should learn how a contracted muscle feels, compared to a relaxed muscle. Sometimes we live with chronic muscular contractions for so long that we forget how normal muscle tone feels. Check which muscles are tense. Look for contractions and pains. If you find any, work more extensively on those muscles.

Yoga exercises are excellent for stretching and relaxing muscles. Yoga also includes breathing exercises. The exercises should not be confused with the yoga philosophy, which instructs on a complete life-style.

Social Prevention

I have traveled enough to see hunger widespread on five continents. In the 1979 book *World Hunger: Ten Myths,* Frances Moore Lappe and Joseph Collius stress that food shortage is a myth but hunger is a reality. We are not growing food for everybody, but only for those selected sectors of the world that can afford higher prices. Grains are grown to feed cattle rather than people to bring high profits to the meat industry. To live with such abundance is immoral. It is more important to ban hunger than pornography. Yet the world remains silent.

A strong economy benefits health care. However, if governments are diseased, health care suffers. An ill government will infect the social structure, and accordingly, society will infect its people.

The World Health Organization has shown that low socioeconomic status is directly related to shorter life expectancy, increased risk for mental disorders, increased risk for cancer, higher infant mortality rate, increase of lung cancer, and increase of high blood pressure.

Important life passages such as moving from adolescence to adulthood or from adulthood to senescence, marriage, economic losses, or having to migrate for work or political reasons may precipitate illnesses such as schizophrenia, tuberculosis, depression, and heart disease. We, as thinking individuals, would do well to be aware that any meaningful change in our social situation may precipitate an illness. Furthermore, psychosocial factors can either maintain or destroy our health.

H. N. Brenner developed equations using unemployment and inflation rates and per capita income to predict several pathological states, such as first admissions to mental hospitals, mortality, suicide, homicide, death from liver cirrhosis (usually related to alcoholism), cardiovascular-renal mortality, and imprisonment. His findings, given in the symposium "Society and Stress" in 1981, were distressing. An increased unemployment rate was significantly associated with increases in each pathology.

Can we not assume, then, that when a government declares that a 10 percent unemployment rate is desirable for a healthy economy, this will be maintained by an unhealthy population?

Is there anything we can do to prevent becoming jobless? On a personal basis, we must keep in mind our good qualities and talents, our interests. We should keep abreast by learning more, developing hobbies, knowing what we enjoy and do best.

Brenner also described the "principle of acceleration," that is, a harmful life change is capable of producing stress, that in turn leads to another life change and subsequent stress. He also established the "principle of contagion," or the effect of one person's stress upon another's. This means an individual may unwillingly transmit not only infectious but emotional disease and maladaptive behavior.

Are we ready to quarantine our homes? Are we ready to single out one member of the family as the black sheep who brings upon us every kind of sickness? Instead, we should practice social prevention. This includes family planning, prenatal and infant care, immunization, control of sexually transmitted diseases, proper nutrition, sanitary housing facilities, and hypertension control.

In the community at large, the main task is to educate those in charge of the various aspects of health care. Ignorance, neglect, inefficiency, red tape, and lack of funds are the main enemies encountered in the struggle to implement a moderately ambitious health project.

No matter how you look at it, preventive medicine can only be achieved in economic terms. We must control our economic greed and redistribute the world's earnings among the vast majority who are not given a chance to eat, let alone become integral beings. How can one think of becoming integral when one can hardly survive? First, we fill our stomachs, then we build a roof over our heads, and thereafter we discuss philosophy.

··· *Chapter Twelve*

WE AND THE BEYOND

> The gorilla, the chimpanzee, the orangutan, and their congener might consider man as a poor and diseased animal that even stores his corpses. And for what?
>
> Miguel de Unamuno,
> *Tragic Sense of Life* (1921)

We must expand our awareness beyond known frontiers to reach new horizons, territories where no visible power can restrain us from our right to search for the universal truth, a truth still veiled for most of us.

Do we have to keep our corpses just in case?

Orthodox religion has failed to explain satisfactorily our presence on this planet, within a material or spiritual context. Eastern and Western philosophies cannot deliver what is not within their grasp. Because each of us perceives a different reality, it is impossible to agree upon evidences of a beyond still unreachable in our modest comprehension.

I have always wondered, if I was on the verge of hallucinating, whether or not I could endure the presence of voices without bodies, or the magic of images of untouchable objects. I question the limits of my rationality and the recurring round-trip to mirrors of questionable replications of what we accept as real or not real. I have suffered having to witness unfinished dreams. I have cherished the absence of dream recall, considering them sometimes too dreadful to remember. I cannot accept that a dream is only an electrobiochemical phenomenon. Instead it is a dash of mystery in my life, a revelation to please or displease my desire to master my fate. I respect the twilight zone of my brain, my fantasies, and the eternal bond that links human beings to this universe forever and for good.

We all need continuity; we secretly hope for a beyond of peace and joy. We are unwilling to accept a return to dust because at the end of our life we will never be satisfied with what we had and what we were. It is very sad to die indifferently, but much worse to die with remorse.

The thoughts and feelings of the integral being could enjoy a longer voyage. To do so we have to awaken the dormant potential of our brains. For an integral being, death is the final new experience.

It took us millions of years to find out that we came from the sea. Our cells, trillions of them, come from one ovule and one sperm. The food we eat, the water we drink, the air we breathe, and the light that shines upon us keep us alive and make us what we are. We are a mixture of history, skin, flesh, bones, intellect, and emotions. The pleasures and burdens of life are all within ourselves.

After seventy years or so of walking, we finally arrive at the end of our life. We look behind and the earth appears the same to us, but we have changed. We are running out of time. Time that belongs only to the human race; a time we wish would never run out for us. Is this all there is?

I remember the priest who was dying, rejecting the idea of the Kingdom of Heaven. I remember the seventeen-year-old girl dying of sclerodermia, who clung to me and asked me not to let her die. As if I were the watchmaker of eternal time and not just a physician patching up pain, bleeding, and despair. I remember the suicidal patient coming out of his coma and cursing me because I interrupted his attempt to end his life. I remember him especially because I met him again five years later and he told me that life was wonderful, when for me life was steadily losing meaning.

We are ready to die. Is my whole life to be packed inside an urn? Should I place it in a coffin underground or in a container neatly stored on the shelf of a mausoleum? How about being laid on the ground as a carcass to feed the birds, to fertilize the earth?

To die, decease, succumb, expire, perish, pass on, meet one's maker, depart, to make one's exit. I like the last one best. To make one's exit to where? Is there something beyond my comprehension? An invisible world for which I will buy new lenses so my mortal blindness will fall away? Once in a while I pinch my skin to be sure I am alive in my own reality. I am thankful then that I am not a solipsist trying to find out whether there is something beyond his other own self.

Is there a beyond, or do we invent one in order to make our transition into death easier?

It is difficult to say with any certainty that yes, there is a beyond. Thousands of individuals, who have been near death and then revived, report having seen either a loved relative or friend just as they thought they were dying. The experience is always described as pleasurable and peaceful, a sensation never sensed when "alive."

Everything we cannot fit within the laws of nature we consider supernatural. Our knowledge and senses limit our understanding and perception of what surrounds us. Nevertheless, we try to explain, by reasoning or faith, whatever occurs in our existence. We have constructed a system of beliefs to protect us in the face of famine, calamity, or war. Toward that end, we began to worship visible objects we believed were in control of our life on earth. The sun, the moon, the wind, the thunderbolt, all became part of primitive religion.

Older civilizations developed the concept of modern religion by substituting visible objects having human or animal characteristics: the gods. Magic—the art of influencing the course of events and of producing phenomena—grew. The purpose of magic and religion was to obtain protection, control the elements, and make wishes come true. In religion, we add the desire to secure a favorable place in a life after death.

The differences between magic and religion are not so significant. Both have a set of common elements, beliefs, and ceremonies. Their main difference is the great number of people practicing organized religion, while magic is a one-to-one experience: the magician and the believer.

When it comes to religion, we have three choices: to profess, to reject, to doubt. These choices are part of our freedom of thought, although they may not be respected by some societies. People have been persecuted, burned, incarcerated, and killed as a consequence of having chosen the "wrong" religion at the wrong time, or having chosen none at all. On behalf of God, many wars have been fought, each side claiming "God is on our side." Assuming that God exists, God cannot be used as a commodity. Religious groups have a mistaken idea about the ownership of God, leading to fighting due to competition rather than righteousness.

With so many political and socioeconomic interests vested in religion today, several faiths are losing spiritual credibility. Why is this happening? Is it because we have developed enough materialism and technology to make spiritual beliefs seem laughable and shameful? Has spiritual belief been undermined by our still precarious knowledge of the universe, or is it because of our failure to trust ourselves?

Because organized religion does not live up to our expectations, we are moving back into witchcraft, the occult, and the worship of the profane. We demand the delivery of what has been promised us and the freedom to exercise our rights. In the meantime, we build up hope for the beyond. The dead, the soul, the angel, the spiritual being, the ghost, whatever is invisible and intangible, beyond our known senses, is awaiting our arrival. This encounter might be arranged by training our extrasensory perception—the closest link between ourselves and the beyond.

Extrasensory perception (ESP), also known as paranormal cognition, is the ability of the brain to function outside its known limits. By using telepathy we may communicate our thoughts, impressions, ideas, or feelings to another brain without the apparent use of our sensorial channels. Or we may use telekinesis to move objects without participation of our physical selves. We may also detect things or events out of our immediate presence, a process known as clairvoyance. There is also precognition, the capacity to know in advance what will occur.

If we utilize other sources of perception, it is certain that our energy will be involved in the mechanism of that perception, since we are atoms that produce energy. If there is energy that emanates from our body to the outside, is it possible to measure or to see it? So far we are able to measure only the electrical impulses of our organs, for instance, the brain or the heart. Many centuries ago, artists in Mediterranean countries and in India painted saints with halos surrounding their bodies. This image reoccurred in the paintings of Christian saints. Did they really see an aura around the holy bodies?

At the beginning of this century, Dr. W. Kilner of London, by using a specially stained glass screen, could observe the aura around a human being. In 1935, two Russian scientists, Semyon Kirilian and his wife, Valentine, were able to photograph energy emanating from the body. They used a high-frequency, high-voltage photographic system that reproduces the electrical field. The energy was manifested as an aura or corona surrounding the body. During an illness, Kirilian photography shows changes in the aura. It also shows different versions of the aura under different weather conditions, the influence of drugs, or hypnotic suggestion. The Kirilian method can be used to photograph other living organisms, including plants and animals. Is the Kirilian effect just an emission of electrical particles, or is it psychic energy?

If this energy exists, what do we do with it? Will it help us to establish communication with the beyond, with other people, as in telepathy, or with other living organisms?

The Aristotelian belief that plants had a soul was accepted until the eighteenth century when Carl Von Linne, known as Linnaeus, published the first monumental work on plant classification. He believed that the only difference between us and plants was the latter's immobility. In 1966, Cleve Backster, an authority on polygraphy for lie-detector systems, placed polygraph electrodes on his office philodendron. He wanted to know how long it would take his plant, just watered, to absorb liquid. To his surprise, he observed a tracing identical to the tracing of humans experiencing emotions. Since then, many experiments have been conducted. It is hard to believe that plants can perceive, but it has been shown that talking lovingly to a plant will make the plant flourish and grow. It has also been shown that threatening a plant will modify its polygraphic tracing.

Another phenomenon that requires further understanding is healing. According to traditional medicine, the healing of wounds takes about seven days. We know that the damage done by illness in many cases can be healed without our conscious intervention, such as the healing of a broken bone, a burn, a stomach ulcer, and so forth. We also know of the use of medication to suppress symptoms such as fever or pain and the use of surgery for other repairs. In the animal kingdom, self-healing is much more evident. Perhaps modern medicine with its discoveries has taken away the self-healing capacity. Is self-healing an automatic act, like the healing of a flesh wound? Or is it the utilization of conscious effort or psychic energy? If we can self-heal ourselves, can we heal others with the power of the mind?

Psychic healers would say yes, although psychic healing is still far from being explained at a scientific level. Of course, the fact that we cannot explain it doesn't automatically rule out its existence. Catholic authorities have appointed medical experts of various religious backgrounds to investigate the occurrence of the miracles that take place at certain shrines like the Virgin of Lourdes in France. On many occasions it has been medically shown that there were no natural medical explanations for the miracles recorded. Among laymen healers, the case of Ardigo, the psychic surgeon of Brazil, is best known. In his operations, Ardigo had complete disregard for anesthesia and the dangers of infection. He operated with fast movements with a pocket knife and finished within minutes. Patients did not report pain and healed well. Ardigo had no knowledge of medicine. He claimed that during his medical tasks the spirit of a deceased German physician possessed him, enabling him to do the job. Ardigo's work was observed by several medical teams, including one from the United States, yet fakery could not be proven.

Some of us may be transmitters or receivers of what is still considered the unknown. The invisible, untouchable, and silent forces that surround us may be available for exploration as we pursue our research.

Is it possible that our thoughts fly away from us and float in the ether with thoughts of other living organisms? Can these thoughts be recaptured by others and recycled and used for good purposes?

Why is the study of the supernatural so weakly supported by official institutions? Are there vested interests that discourage the study of the supernatural? Will discoveries in this area upset traditional religious beliefs?

Could discoveries in the area of the supernatural facilitate the birth of a true, free integral being?

Could the supernatural shake the structures of world power, shifting this power to its natural recipient—us? What sociopolitical changes would take place if we walk into the beyond?

To my dismay, I read recently that representatives of some of the largest corporations held meetings to discuss how metaphysics, the occult, and Hindu mysticism might help executives to compete in the world market.

Will knowledge of the supernatural be used for good or for ill?

We are free to reach our own conclusions.

••• *Chapter Thirteen*

THE ONGOING YOU

> The moment the slave resolves that he will no longer be a slave, his fetters fall. He frees himself and shows the way to others. Freedom and slavery are neutral states.
>
> Mohandas K. Gandhi,
> *Non-Violence in Peace and War* (1948)

Now we should consider the idea of becoming an integral being. To assume an integral life-style requires a serious analysis of what is convenient and suitable to our needs and how much freedom is available. Life-style is determined by our upbringing as children, our trade or profession, and, always, by our economic resources. Most of the time, life-style choice takes place when we are ready to leave home.

Can we change our life-style to an integral one? As long as we have the will to change, it is never too late for changes.

Let us consider the ongoing you. Ultimately you will have to free yourself of undesirable habits, attitudes, and behaviors that are obstacles to becoming integral. So let us review the major determinants in life-style: sex, love, work, and success.

•••

Sex

Sexual organs are visible or concealed anatomy, physical realities utilized to distinguish men from women. To paraphrase Descartes, I have a vagina, therefore I am a woman; I have a penis, therefore I am a man. Sex is not, however, merely anatomical differences. Gender has been used to assign social roles, partly determined by factors such as muscular strength in men and childbearing ability in women. In the struggle for power between the sexes, men monopolized education. The long history of deprivation of women's rights can be traced to a lack of education. Until very recently, women were not allowed to learn to read and write. Therefore, women were systematically prevented from entering the worlds of philosophy, science, business, and the arts. Myths developed: men are physically stronger, harder workers, and sexually free; women are physically weaker, passive, spiritually inclined, and sexually inhibited.

If both sexes had had equal opportunities for growth and education, great psychological, social, and behavioral differences would not have developed. The existing differences between the sexes have been imposed and learned throughout the centuries. Women and men are not born with psychological or behavioral differences. Babies do not choose pink or blue, dolls or trucks, baseball or ballet. These so-called choices are impositions; in reality, we are all expected to behave, dress, perform, and even choose trades according to social expectations. These differences should be erased because they advocate and perpetuate women's slavery. We risk embarrassment as individuals preaching freedom when freedom is not fully shared by women.

As a consequence of women's oppression, men have had access to an endless source of information enabling them to control the administration of countries, to become leading scientists, teachers, and artisans. Men have become intellectually richer, capable of being better thinkers, creators, and executives. By allowing men to have all the advantages, society reinforced the concept that man is better than woman. The woman becomes a second-class citizen, a slave, or, to put it nicely, "She's only a housewife." A woman's mission is to beget and raise children and take care of the house. Hence, there is no need for women to have access to the world.

Nevertheless, a female labor force is growing rapidly worldwide. From blue-collar jobs to high public office, women are playing an important role. In Africa, 80 percent of the farming is operated by women.

Let us fix in our minds that except for our physical differences, we are all the same. To support any other belief is to sponsor a myth and to promote slavery.

When we were little children we were told not to play with our genitals. Our genitals had funny nicknames, perhaps to allow us to avoid the shame of using real names. Masturbation was believed to cause mental retardation, or it was sinful. Masturbation still produces guilt and embarrassment for many who practice it. There is nothing obscene or sinful about masturbation, but there is something quite wrong with the social attitude that condemns it.

We grow up sexually troubled, burdened by feelings of guilt about sex. Usually it is introduced to us surrounded by shame, fear, and punishment. Sex is a dirty word for those who preach abstinence, a burden for inhibited wives, a chore for money-making men, a disorder for the psychoanalyst, and a profitable item for entrepreneurs. Sex is looked at as a curse, a disease, a commercial product, or as a sin, rarely as a loving and sharing experience.

Parents, educators, religious leaders, communities, and governments have double standards in explaining their attitudes toward sex. How many laws against sexual acts exist? On the other hand, why does the mass media promote so much sex to sell jeans? Double standards conflict us. Double standards enable us to use women as sex symbols, deprived of intelligence and dignity. Furthermore, the combination of violence and sex offered by the media teaches our children to view sex as an aggressive act.

Most of us will have sexual intercourse with the opposite sex. Should we reject our sexual anatomy and prefer a different sexual identity based on an emotional need, society will reject us. If society restricts sex even among consenting adults, imagine what it does to homosexuals. Homosexuality is neither a disease nor immoral, but a social conflict. When we make the choice to become sexually active, we assume responsibility for it. I am not advocating promiscuity, but freedom for individuals to decide how they will express their sexuality.

The human sexual response is much more than a biological and instinctual response. It is the giving of the entire self to another human being. If we want to know how good a sexual partner we are, let's ask our mate. It saves time and sorrow.

If sexual difficulties exist, they may be due to other problems in the relationship. Economic difficulties, disagreement on life-style, and undefined goals as a couple can end up causing sexual trouble. An important cause of sexual difficulties is self-centeredness. Egotistical persons can rarely share in sex because they only take.

For the integral being, sex is beauty and mystery. We don't have to be scientific about everything; we can savor living with mysterious things. If we sit back and think of it, the sexual act is a secret that we may share with those whom we love.

Love

What is love for you? I can ask the question, but I won't be able to answer it because love is the most secret emotion of all. The recipient of your love will know about your loving behavior, but will never know what your love is. This private emotion, steady or unstable, certain or doubtful, brands your emotional being with its own character. A character that only you can modify. There is a positive yet symbiotic connection between love and the ongoing you. True love is wholesome and promotes the equilibrium between you, nature, and the universe. Love is one of the emotions the ongoing you will never suppress in order to become an integral being.

But, again, what is love for you? A feeling that changes very often? An emotion that hardly surfaces? Do you see love as a very deep sharing experience with someone you like? Are there different kinds of love? Love of parents, spouses, lovers, children, relatives, friends, land, arts, and so forth? Or is love one single emotion divided among those whom you love? What is love for you?

Work

Most of us do not work in the area of our real interests. This regrettable situation affects people from many different socioeconomic backgrounds. At a certain point in our life, each of us either wants or needs to work. Educating ourselves for the labor market may take a few months to several years of study, depending on the degree of difficulty in attaining the necessary skills. Many of us may choose a particular career in order to preserve family tradition, to fulfill the dreams of parents, to make a good income, or, sometimes, to satisfy our own desires.

Too often we are forced to let money dictate our choice of work. When we are in need of money to support our families and ourselves, we capitulate. This capitulation and loss of freedom on economic grounds will result in the most serious conflict for the ongoing you.

As a psychiatrist, and as an individual, I am always meeting people who eventually admit lack of interest in their work. Many of these people are successful and wealthy; they would love a second opportunity to do what they really want to do.

Will remaining in an unwanted job interfere with becoming an integral being? As long as we do our best to remain free, it will not interfere with our program to become an integral being. We may be bound to our work from nine to five, but we can pursue our own interests the rest of the time.

At some point, we may decide to succeed within ourselves, growing in the dimension of spiritual tolerance and peace. This may enhance our program to become an integral being. We will use parameters alien to the world of consumerism and material success, developing values that will not purchase merchandise but are ways to integrate ourselves with the universe.

Success

To succeed is to work toward or accomplish goals. Teamwork is required of our body, intellect, and emotional resources.

Society looks at success through an economic lens; mastering the art of living or the art of loving is not considered a success. Those who make it economically are viewed as successful. It doesn't matter what means were employed to become wealthy, society has its way of redefining the word *moral* so as to excuse immorality. This is because money goes hand in hand with power, the ultimate combination for a successful person. Each day the media provides us with stories of success viewed in terms of money and power. It would be far more valuable to teach that success is health, love, and work, things not easily achieved.

Are we born to success? No one is, but we are given the tools to achieve it: our body, emotions, and intellect. If these tools are not kept in shape, we are destined to fail.

To succeed, we first have to educate ourselves. Knowledge, sacrifice, discipline, and perseverance are forms of success. We ought to know what we want out of life. Too many people are adrift, unwilling to commit themselves. They want everything here and now, with little personal effort. They allow circumstances and others to rule their lives.

Is it important that we succeed? We must first decide what success is for us. Is it the money-power idea? Is it to develop ourselves as integral beings? Or is it both? When we know what success means to us, then we must ask ourselves whether or not we want to succeed. Is it worth it to succeed? Do we do it for ourselves or for others?

Finally, we get the message: we must succeed. We have to become integral beings; any other kind of success is welcome, but not indispensable.

♦ ♦ ♦

The Journey

As the Peace Pilgrim said, "I am a pilgrim, a wanderer. I shall remain a wanderer until mankind has learned the way to peace, walking until I am given shelter and fasting until I am given food."

I have shown you a crumbling world, full of political deceit, famine, injustice, and the horror of torture and war. However, there is also a world out there of hope, of discoveries, of great individuals who dedicate their lives to the progress of mankind.

These two worlds compete for supremacy. Today there is a serious gap between them, a gap caused by good and evil—the natural polarizing forces of life. Perhaps the world was before as it is today and it will be tomorrow. Our world may not change the course of the universe, but certainly it changes ours. The integral being's task is to build the bridge, so we can cross it in both directions, so we can bring both worlds together into one single world of peace.

You are alone. From the time of your birth you carry within yourself a loneliness that will never leave you. When all our oldest relatives die, the witnesses of our birth also die. At this point in our life, we develop full awareness of our loneliness. There is another loneliness, a social loneliness that we dwell in if we choose. You look at yourself in the mirror to observe the rhythmic expansion of your chest. You decide to hold your breath and it is possible. You see it as a funny event and you smile. You try some ballet steps and you become excited by your laughing, your movements, your sounds. Finally you get tired and rest. Now you are aware that you can master your body, you can rule, you can do and even undo.

But you are frightened of this discovery of your powers.

You look back on your life and see how much you did and how much you didn't. Only you have the responsibility for your own growth, to make choices and decisions. You have a brain, the knowledge, the feelings, the sense of duty, and all those passions trying to break through the barricade of norms, laws, ignorance, and stagnation.

You are still in your room in front of the mirror, afraid to go out and face the world. You look at your bed, wishing it was a crib. It would be nice to be a baby again. Yes, you love to be nurtured and cared for. But now you are of age. We cannot play house forever—or can we? Do you expect to see someone else in the mirror? Another you?

When you came to this earth you were a small triangle of body, intellect, and emotions surrounded by the big triangle of government, society, and family. Both triangles were placed inside the square of nature, and all of it inside the circle of the universe. You must adjust to these relationships. It can be done.

The flame of an integral being is already inside you. The spark of your life lighted long ago, beyond the scope of our own universe. Keep the flame within yourself; outside it will be blown and threatened with extinguishment by the world.

Wherever you go, you cannot get away from yourself. You have no excuse to procrastinate, to delay, or to alter your desire to become an integral being. But to become an integral being, your presence on this earth has to be meaningful to you. Without a meaning, you cannot have a lasting motivation. You must find a meaning that will live within you wherever you go, whatever you do. Even imprisoned, you must find a meaning to your presence. Otherwise, everything becomes hopeless, destructive, and overwhelming. You have to learn to be alone with yourself.

You have to love yourself and accept what is good in you and change what you dislike. Because in the end it is up to you to be or not to be, to have or not to have, to do or not to do, to become or to vanish.

Your decision will be a turning point in your life. As I have repeated to myself so many times: What I think is not what I imagine, and what I imagine is not what I feel.

EPILOGUE

I am now ready to close this book. I worry whether I have been able to convey successfully the idea that without harmony among us and the universe, our family, society, and government, health cannot be kept and life becomes miserable. The interaction among all those factors is profound; it is a magnetic force that keeps us all orbiting together.

While writing this book, I tried more than ever to put into practice—should I say it?—what I preach, and believe me, it is hard!

One is frightened, at times hopeful. On other occasions enthusiasm floods our senses, and the mind flies high and strong. Then there is the frustration, the constant struggle, the realization that this world is being systematically raped by those, invested by force and deceit, who are our rulers and unwanted prophets.

I go to the mirror and I look at myself, and I read the front page and I listen to the news and I see the curiosity of children and the glimpse of dreams in young people, and I listen and talk to my patients and I faithfully write my poetry and systematically become anxious when I go for my physical checkup.

Everything wrinkles, including the pages of this book. But who will give up? I won't!

OCT - 5 199